Praise for
Wake Up to Sleep

'Healthcare providers as well as insomniacs will discover
how to combine powerful techniques including
mindfulness, breathing and lucid dreaming illustrated by
poignant examples from Charlie's work with veterans.'

DR PATRICIA GERBARG, CO-AUTHOR OF THE HEALING POWER
OF THE BREATH AND ASSISTANT PROFESSOR IN CLINICAL
PSYCHIATRY, NEW YORK MEDICAL COLLEGE

'Learning from Charlie felt like him taking me by the hand
and guiding me on an exploration of my own mind. I highly
recommend him not only for his knowledge of the subject
matter but more so for his unique ability to teach in a fun
and compelling way that gets results for his students.'

VISHEN LAKHIANI, NEW YORK TIMES BESTSELLING AUTHOR
AND FOUNDER OF MINDVALLEY

'This is a highly informative book from a deep and
authentic teacher. These practices can make a big difference
to sleep and mental wellbeing. I anticipate that this
book will help a great many people who struggle with
sleep and I will recommend it to my own patients.'

DR HEATHER SEQUERIA PHD, CHARTERED PSYCHOLOGIST

'Wake Up to Sleep illustrates brilliantly the nuts and bolts of
why and how to self-regulate our autonomic nervous system
to achieve healthy sleep and enhance our wellbeing, and at
the same time conveys the sacred nature of the endeavour.'

GARRET YOUNT PHD, MOLECULAR NEUROBIOLOGIST,
INSTITUTE OF NOETIC SCIENCES

'I wish I had access to this kind of stuff
when I returned from Afghanistan.'

S. WILLIAMSON, NAVAL OFFICER WITH 45 COMMANDO ROYAL MARINES

'Charlie gives us the science and the know-how to
help integrate trauma, calm the nervous system,
breathe better and sleep soundly. This is a book to
refer to time and time again for years to come.'

DR DAVID HAMILTON, BESTSELLING AUTHOR OF
HOW YOUR MIND CAN HEAL YOUR BODY

'This book should be required reading for anyone
seeking to help people suffering from the symptoms
of post-traumatic stress. If you're struggling with
insomnia, this book could change your life.'

MATTHEW GREEN, AUTHOR OF AFTERSHOCK: FIGHTING
WAR, SURVIVING TRAUMA AND FINDING PEACE

'Everyone falls in love with Charlie's work. Why? Because
it exudes love. And just when you think he has levelled out,
he produces his most powerful work yet. I would advise
everyone, whatever their walk of life, to read this book for I
guarantee it will allow you to change your life dramatically.'

KEITH MCKENZIE, PARATROOPER VETERAN AND BUDDHIST CHAPLAIN

Also by Charlie Morley

<u>Books</u>

Lucid Dreaming Made Easy (2018)

Dreaming Through Darkness (2017)

Dreams of Awakening (2013)

<u>Audio downloads</u>

Lucid Dreaming Made Easy (2018)

Dreaming Through Darkness (2017)

Dreams of Awakening (2017)

Lucid Dreaming, Conscious Sleeping (2015)

<u>Online courses</u>

Lucid Dreaming (2015)

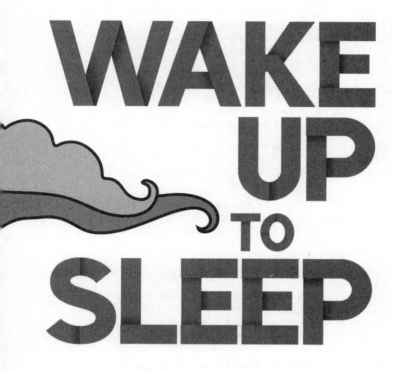

WAKE UP TO SLEEP

5 POWERFUL PRACTICES
TO TRANSFORM STRESS & TRAUMA
FOR PEACEFUL SLEEP & MINDFUL DREAMS

CHARLIE MORLEY

HAY HOUSE

Carlsbad, California • New York City
London • Sydney • New Delhi

Published in the United Kingdom by:
Hay House UK Ltd, The Sixth Floor, Watson House,
54 Baker Street, London W1U 7BU
Tel: +44 (0)20 3927 7290; Fax: +44 (0)20 3927 7291; www.hayhouse.co.uk

Published in the United States of America by:
Hay House Inc., PO Box 5100, Carlsbad, CA 92018-5100
Tel: (1) 760 431 7695 or (800) 654 5126
Fax: (1) 760 431 6948 or (800) 650 5115; www.hayhouse.com

Published in Australia by:
Hay House Australia Pty Ltd, 18/36 Ralph St, Alexandria NSW 2015
Tel: (61) 2 9669 4299; Fax: (61) 2 9669 4144; www.hayhouse.com.au

Published in India by:
Hay House Publishers India, Muskaan Complex,
Plot No.3, B-2, Vasant Kunj, New Delhi 110 070
Tel: (91) 11 4176 1620; Fax: (91) 11 4176 1630; www.hayhouse.co.in

A catalogue record for this book is available from the British Library.

Tradepaper ISBN: 978-1-4019-6321-7
E-book ISBN: 978-1-78817-627-9
Audiobook ISBN: 978-1-78817-624-8

10 9 8 7 6 5 4 3 2 1

Printed in the United States of America

For Keith McKenzie and all those who've served.

Contents

PART III: AND BREATHE...

PART IV: NIGHTMARE INTEGRATION

PART V: LUCID DREAMING

List of Exercises

Dr Sunil M. Kariyakarawana
B.A. honours. (Kel), M.A. (Ottawa) PhD (Cornell)
Buddhist Civilian Chaplain to the Military
Chaplains Branch
Headquarters London District

ARMY

Foreword

Living in the third decade of the 21st century with all its scientific and technological advancements, humanity is navigating an exciting phase with regards to the 'outside world'. With regards to our 'inside world' though, we still do not seem to know very much!

This reminds me of an ancient tale, which says that while roaming around the Himalayas, a powerful deity found the 'secret of happiness' for all mankind but out of jealousy wanted to hide it from humans. He asked himself: *Should I hide it at the top of a Himalayan mountain? Or should I hide it at the bottom of the deepest ocean?* He finally concluded that the best place to hide anything from humans would be to place it 'just below their own nose', since they would search everywhere in the outside world before searching within themselves.

It was indeed the historical Buddha himself, the 'extraordinary human' who discovered that 'the secret of happiness lies just below one's own nose, and one's own breath is a gateway to one's own heart and mind.'

Drawing from such ancient wisdom and testing it against modern scientific research, Charlie has been developing his Mindfulness of Dream & Sleep approach for many years now. As a young researcher and committed Buddhist practitioner, he has been specializing in this area from both theoretical and practical perspectives. Charlie's work with both veterans and serving members of the British Armed Forces has taken his research to new heights, and its impact has been quite groundbreaking and positively received.

3-Star General and Diversity Champion Lt. General Robert Magowan (who also leads the Defence Mindfulness Steering Group) has been admiring Charlie's work throughout:

> *'Charlie's pioneering Mindfulness of Dream & Sleep work has already delivered great results within the UK Defence community. Undoubtedly, the techniques and approaches he advocates will continue to be of interest and use to serving members of Defence forces, who are expected to show best behaviour in the worst of circumstances. I am hugely grateful to Charlie for the work he has already done and I know will continue to do.'*
>
> LT. GENERAL RA MAGOWAN CB, CBE
> DEPUTY COMMANDER UK STRATEGIC COMMAND AND COMMANDANT
> GENERAL ROYAL MARINES

The five main practices that Charlie explores in this book have been well researched and are textually supported by the ancient Buddhist wisdom and insights found in the Pāli canon. The third of the five practices – Coherent Breathing –

has been specifically mentioned by the Buddha himself in the Mindfulness of Breathing Sutra as the fourth ('tranquilizing the breath') of the 16 stages in the path to enlightenment.

As the first ever Buddhist spiritual caregiver to over 5,000 serving Buddhists in the British Armed Forces for the past 16 years, I can confidently say that young Charlie has a lot to offer, not just to the Defence community but to the whole of humanity, especially at this time when we find ourselves at a crossroads for global mental health and wellbeing.

Sunil Kariyakarawana PhD
Buddhist Chaplain to Her Majesty's British Armed Forces
Director, Kalyana Mitra: Buddhist Chaplaincy
  Support Group

Introduction

I was 17 when I first experienced how trauma can affect sleep.

I was coming to the end of a wild time of drugs, gangs and all-night raves that would eventually lead me to the spiritual path, but not before a game-changing final initiation. An accidentally large dose of psychedelics led to a full-on near-death experience that left me with panic attacks, nightmares and flashbacks – all the hallmarks of what I can now see was most probably PTSD.

After months of recurring nightmares, it was my burgeoning practice of lucid dreaming (becoming conscious in a dream and directing the dream at will) that eventually integrated them, and my new practice of mindfulness that calmed the daytime panics.

Since then I've spent a large part of my life learning, sharing and building on those dreamwork and mindfulness practices that saved me from losing my mind 20 years ago. I formally became a Buddhist at the age of 19 and ended up living in the

London Samye Dzong Buddhist centre for seven years and writing three books on dreamwork and Shadow integration.

I started teaching sleep and dream practices professionally in 2008, and I soon found that more and more people working with nightmares and trauma were turning up at the workshops. In many cases, the techniques they learned helped to reduce or often completely integrate their nightmares, but I also noticed that there was another crucial factor at play too: shared experience. My own first-hand knowledge of trauma nightmares seemed to help people to trust that the practices that I was offering could and would work. There was the kind of mutual kinship that you only feel when you meet someone who has known a similar pain. You can see it in each other's eyes and you often share a look that says, 'You too? Yeah, I know that place.'

At a retreat that I was running in 2013 I met a man named Keith McKenzie. As he told me about his nightmares, I felt that familiar kinship, but as I looked into his eyes, I realized that this time I didn't 'know that place'. And no wonder: Keith was a veteran of the British army's Parachute Regiment as well as a retired firefighter with 20 years' service. He had been to places that I could never know.

Keith had quite a breakthrough at that retreat, as he was able to, in his words, 'integrate more of my PTSD in that four-day retreat than in four years of therapy'.

A few years later, when Keith had become a fully trained mindfulness meditation teacher and armed forces Buddhist chaplain, he asked me if I would come to one of the mindfulness retreats that he had organized for military veterans and teach them the same techniques.

I had no idea whether the sleep and dream techniques that had worked for Keith would work for other veterans, but I was keen to try. From the off, I knew that when working with veterans, the goals would be very different from when working with civilians. Our main focus would be on sleeping better and integrating nightmares. No complex lucid dreaming techniques or esoteric Buddhist theory, just a simple focus on sleeping soundly and safely.

The most common ways of working with troubled sleep are to change either the symptoms through medication or the external conditions through sleep hygiene. Both of these are like changing the weather but not changing the climate.[1] For people who *are not* experiencing high levels of stress or trauma, this might work quite well. But for those who were, I realized, it was necessary to change the actual climate of their sleep rather than just help them weather the current storm.

The sleep and dream practices worked well and most of the veterans benefitted from them. Even those who didn't connect so much with them did find deep relief in the breath and bodywork practices that the trauma-informed yoga and *chi gong* teachers were offering on the retreat. So I saw that those practices were just as important for regulating sleep as the ones that I was offering.

The veterans' retreats touched me deeply. Some of the stories the veterans told and the nightmares they shared will be forever etched on my memory. Those men and women bore their scars with a courage and dignity I hadn't dreamed possible.

Inspired by that first retreat, I began working with more veterans' groups and then with serving military personnel too. In 2018 this led me to secure a Winston Churchill Memorial Trust Fellowship to research best practice in mindfulness-based approaches to PTSD. The research took me to the USA and Canada to study and train with some of the leading organizations in the field, such as iRest Yoga Nidra and Breath-Body-Mind, both of which impressed me so much that I ended up taking their teacher training courses.

When I added these deep relaxation, breath and bodywork practices to the lucid dreaming and mindfulness practices that I was already teaching, it became clear that a very effective five-part programme was starting to emerge. When I ran that programme, 'Mindfulness of Dream & Sleep', with veterans working with PTSD, and later with civilians, we started to see some impressive results. So much so that in 2019 I was asked to present my findings at a mindfulness symposium taking place at the UK Ministry of Defence in London. It was quite a bizarre experience to be speaking about lucid dreaming, breathwork and Yoga Nidra to an audience of over 250 military and defence personnel, but the talk was well received and led to further opportunities.

Mental health issues among British armed forces have risen by over two-thirds in the past decade, and as you might imagine, the military is keen to find ways to counteract this. So, on the two 'Mindfulness of Dream & Sleep' live online courses that I ran in 2020, I commissioned an independent report to quantify the effectiveness of the techniques.

Over 140 people took part, two-thirds of whom were military veterans or serving personnel, and one-third civilians struggling with sleep. By the end of the six-week programme, the independent report showed that 87 per cent reported significantly improved sleep quality, while 77 per cent reported significantly lowered levels of anxiety around sleep.[2]

On the first of these courses, 73 per cent of participants reported one or more lucid dreams during the six-week period, while 70 per cent reported a 'large reduction' in the frequency of their nightmares.

These groups contained many people with severe PTSD, so it was becoming clear that the five core practices were a highly effective combination for treating stress or trauma-affected sleep, even in the most heavily traumatized populations. It is those practices that form the basis of this book.

Mindfulness of Dream & Sleep

This term was originally created by the mindfulness pioneer Rob Nairn to describe the holistic approach to lucid dreaming that we created together back in 2008. It now refers to an enthusiastically destigmatizing 'body-based' approach to stress or trauma-affected sleep based around five foundational practices that include breathwork, nightmare integration, deep relaxation and sleep awareness alongside those original lucid dreaming practices.

Each 'foundation' focuses on practical exercises rather than complicated theory, and each technique has been chosen because both scientific research and the results I have witnessed at workshops have shown it to be one of the most effective available.

Each part of this book explores one of the five foundations:

- Part I: Sleep Awareness (learning how sleep works)

- Part II: Rest and Relaxation (practising hypnagogic mindfulness and Yoga Nidra)

- Part III: And Breathe... (regulating and optimizing the nervous system through the breath)

- Part IV: Nightmare Integration (reframing and transforming trauma-affected dreams)

- Part V: Lucid Dreaming (healing trauma through conscious dreaming practices)

Although originally developed for military veterans, the practices in this book have been adapted to be suitable for anyone with stressed-out sleep, and I've seen millennial hipsters gain as much from them as Vietnam vets. Also, since my personal life fell apart at the end of 2019 (a terminal diagnosis for my mum, the end of a 10-year relationship with my wife and a newly broken heart), I've seen first hand how they help with anxiety, insomnia, nightmares and depression.

In fact, the publication of this book got pushed back almost a year as I worked through the heartbreak and depression caused by my mum's rapid decline into Alzheimer's and the end of my marriage. In some ways it was a blessing, though: who was I to write about trauma-affected sleep when I hadn't experienced it for almost 20 years? Of course, what I've been through is incomparable with what so many of the veterans or sexual-abuse survivors I've worked with have been through, but I got at least a reminder of how trauma wreaks havoc upon our nervous system and how these practices help to regulate it.

So, the reason I'm so confident that the practices in this book work is because I personally *know* that they work, not only for clinical PTSD, but also for the more commonplace traumas of familial loss and heartbreak.

A Book Born in Lockdown

Although I've been teaching the practices in this book for several years, it was during the covid-19 lockdowns of 2020 that I wrote the majority of it. Over that time sleep disturbances started to skyrocket and every few weeks I would receive another email from another journalist looking for someone to explain why so many people were reporting anxiety dreams and nightmares.

It was then that I realized that the statistics that told of 60 million people in the USA suffering from one or more clinical sleep disorders[3] and stressed-out sleep affecting 30 per cent of the adult population[4] were collated *before* 2020. As the global trauma of covid-19 and the devastating effects of the lockdowns on mental health start to take effect, we can assume that those figures will get much, much higher.

One of the most beneficial aspects of the 'Mindfulness of Dream & Sleep' programme is that it not only offers an effective long-term approach to healing trauma-affected sleep, but also has a remarkable impact on lowering daytime stress and anxiety levels. The main focus of many of the techniques in this book is on regulating the dysregulated nervous system that stress and trauma create. This dysregulation is a major factor in not only most sleep problems, but in many depression and anxiety-related conditions too.

And as an estimated 80 per cent[5] of chronic insomnia occurs in connection with a so-called psychiatric disorder, all the techniques in this book (with the possible exception of the lucid dreaming ones in Chapter 15) are totally safe for people of all levels of 'mental healthiness'.

Having said that, the aim of this book isn't to fix anyone. We don't need fixing, because we aren't broken. We might be stressed out, or traumatized, or overwhelmed by the weight of chronic anxiety, but we are not broken.

We might be feeling cracked, though… and in that case, just like the Japanese concept of *kintsukuroi*, or 'golden repair' (the art of repairing broken pottery with a resin made with powdered gold), our cracks, rather than being seen as faults, can be embraced as opportunities to re-seal ourselves with precious gold, allowing each healed wound to add to our value rather than detract from it.

And so it is my heart's desire that this book helps you learn how to use your body, breath, sleep and dreams to heal from trauma and integrate anxiety. And that these practices help you to transform not only the third of your life that you spend asleep, but the two-thirds that you spend awake too.

With love and lucidity,

Charlie Morley
Tibetan New Year, 12 February 2021, London

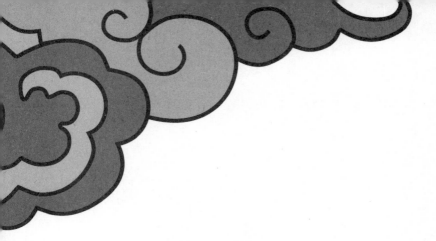

PART I

SLEEP AWARENESS

*'Sleep is the golden chain that ties
health and our bodies together.'*

THOMAS DEKKER, 16TH-CENTURY WRITER

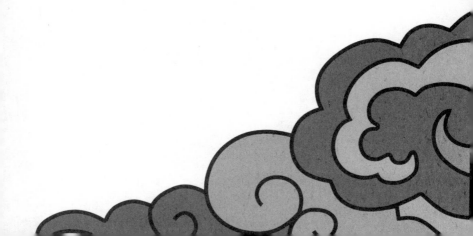

In this first part of the book we'll be exploring how sleep works, how stress and trauma affect it and, crucially, how becoming aware of how we currently sleep is the first step in changing our relationship to it.

CHAPTER 1

A Third of Our Life

'Sleep is the best meditation.'
HH Dalai Lama

Sleep is really, really good for us. We are better at literally everything we can measure when we get sufficient sleep. Sufficient sleep means sleeping for about 30 years, approximately a third of our life.

Of course, this is speculation based on the average lifespan. And yet, interestingly, sleep itself can be used to accurately predict how long we're going to live, because in almost all cases, the shorter our sleep, the shorter our life. This book, though, might just add an extra couple of years to it.

Matthew Walker, Professor of Neuroscience and Psychology at the University of California, Berkeley, and author of the seminal *Why We Sleep*, believes that sleep is the greatest performance-enhancing drug there is and explains that if there were a pill that could make us 30 per cent better at any newly learned skill, while also giving us more creativity, more cognitive ability and more psychological tolerance, we'd be queuing up to buy it.[1] There is such a thing, but it's not a pill, it's a habit – the habit of getting more sleep than usual.

Insufficient sleep, now classed by the National Sleep Foundation as fewer than seven hours per night,[2] leads to measurable cognitive impairment, and there is no biological function in the body that is not adversely affected by it.

Poor sleep affects every part of our life, from cognitive ability – a sleepless night leads to 40 per cent less memory storage[3] – to weight loss – dieting while sleep-deprived loses muscle, not fat.[4]

Even immune function is affected, as we have a whopping 70 per cent drop in immune cell activity after a night of poor sleep.[5] As the late, great sleep pioneer Dr William Dement famously said, 'You're not healthy unless your sleep is healthy.'[6]

Insufficient sleep affects wider society, too, with sleep deprivation being directly linked to tens of thousands of traffic accident deaths every year and to a 170 per cent increase in major surgical error.[7] It even affects the global economy, with over 2 per cent of America's entire GDP – hundreds of billions of dollars – lost each year to illnesses linked to insufficient sleep.[8]

It's Not All Bad

Let's not wallow too much in the misery of how bad poor sleep is for us, though. Instead, let's learn how to transform it into better sleep.

Research from the US National Sleep Foundation (based upon a review of 320 research articles) concluded that adults should aim for a daily dose of seven to nine hours of sleep,[9] but let's be realistic… If you are currently averaging only four or five hours of sleep per night, is this book really going to get you up to nine? Probably not, but it may well get you up to seven, and just an hour or two of extra sleep has been proven to have profound effects on our body and mind. Research from the American Psychological Association found that just 60–90 minutes of extra sleep per night can make us significantly healthier and happier.[10]

It can save lives, too. Fascinatingly, each year when the clocks go back for Daylight Saving and 1.6 billion people across 70 countries gain an extra hour in bed, there is a 21 per cent decrease in heart attacks the next day.[11] There's also a big drop in suicides and car crashes worldwide.[12] That all adds up to tens of thousands of fewer deaths around the world from just one extra hour of sleep.

As we'll learn in Chapter 6, that extra hour doesn't necessarily have to come at night, either. Although seven to nine hours per night should still be aimed for, an hour's nap during the daytime can have powerful effects and may, for some, be a much more realistic way of boosting their overall sleep quota than trying to do it all at night.

~ *Sleep Notes* ~

A well-timed nap can work wonders. A University of California study found that a 90-minute afternoon nap actually led to the same improvement in neurological functioning as a full night's sleep![13] This means that the day after a bad night's sleep doesn't have to be a write-off if you can find time for a sneaky hour or so of shut-eye.

The Sleep Delusion

As recently as 20 years ago it used to be thought that the amount of sleep that each of us needed was pretty subjective: if we had plenty of energy throughout the day and didn't have too much 'brain fog', then we were getting enough sleep. Nowadays, though, neurobiological research has shown that people's subjective opinion of how much sleep they *think* they need is a terrible predictor of how much sleep they *actually* need.[14]

Although many people believe that they function perfectly well on five or six hours' sleep, when scientists test their responsiveness and levels of mental acuity, they find that they are clearly in a state of sub-optimal neurological functioning. The tests clearly show how badly their brains are working, yet they report feeling fine.

What does this mean? It means, tragically, that we have been sleep-deprived for so long that 'sub-optimal neurological functioning' has become our new normal. We have become so habituated to chronic sleep deprivation that our normal 'I feel fine' state has become one of sleep-deprived cognitive impairment. We believe that this is just how we are and so unknowingly resign ourselves to it.

Sleep expert Dr Willam Dement often referenced experiments in which healthy volunteers were paid to stay in bed for 14 hours a day for seven days straight. The results showed that most people were so *unknowingly sleep-deprived* that given the opportunity to do so, they slept for about 12 hours a night for the first few days and then settled into a regular seven to nine hours per night.[15]

Dr Dement concluded: 'Sadly, millions of us are living a less than optimal life and performing at a less than optimal level, impaired by an amount of sleep debt that we're not even aware we carry.'[16]

But what about those of us who go to work, play sports, have a social life and achieve great things while getting just six hours a night?

Exactly, so imagine what you could achieve if you got seven or eight.

Research shows that when five-to-six-hour sleepers start regularly getting just one extra hour, they become more effective at work, more socially proactive, markedly healthier and measurably happier in most areas of life.[17]

Some report feeling that they've tapped into a supercharged state, yet this is actually their totally normal state, but one that insufficient sleep had kept at bay for so long that they'd forgotten it existed.

Mindfulness

The 'Mindfulness of Dream & Sleep' programme that makes up the main body of this book is based on five foundations: sleep awareness; rest and relaxation; breathwork; nightmare integration; and lucid dreaming. All of these have mindfulness at their core, but what does mindfulness actually mean?

Mindfulness is a quality of mind that knows *what* is happening *as* it is happening. It is intentional awareness of the present moment.

Mindfulness, in and of itself, is great for lessening stress and trauma, because when awareness is present, the mind naturally comes into focus and balance. This balance then allows any stressed-out or traumatized aspects of the mind to be gradually reintegrated – something they can and will do naturally when the mind is full of awareness.

Although many people find that sitting in silence and watching their breath is one of the easiest ways to practise mindfulness, that particular practice will be conspicuously absent from this book. This is because it might not be the best choice for someone currently working with trauma. Although it might be fine for many, psychology expert Dr Tobias-Mortlock warns, 'Sitting in silence for 20 minutes may, in traumatized populations, unearth latent trauma in unexpected ways, making them particularly vulnerable.'[18]

Also, with dissociation (a feeling of disconnection from our body or the world around us) being such a common feature in people working with high levels of stress or trauma, I believe that before we drop into our mind, we first need to learn how to drop into our body.

So, body-focused mindfulness practices such as Yoga Nidra (a form of meditative deep relaxation usually done lying down) and Breath-Body-Mind (a collection of breathing techniques combined with mindful movements) are much safer for people working with trauma, while offering the same neurological benefits as standard mindfulness meditation.[19]

And finally, I know this may sound sacrilegious, but as someone who lived in a Tibetan Buddhist centre for over seven years, I can speak from experience: standard mindfulness is just a bit, well, *boring* for most people and so they don't tend to keep it up for long. So, although I am a huge fan of mindfulness, we won't actually be doing much of the sitting-in-silence type.

A Body-Based Approach

The usual approach to stress and trauma is what is known as 'top down': we talk about it with a therapist, which allows us to understand what is going on inside us and helps to process the memories of the trauma. The basic theory, first formulated in the late 1800s, is that by talking about the traumatic experience in detail, within the safe space of the therapeutic dyad, our mind can begin to rationalize and release the painful memories of it.

This kind of 'talking therapy' can be a godsend for many people (as it was for me when my personal life fell apart a couple of years ago), and with so many sleep problems being caused by general stresses and worries (money, relationships, career), it can have a profoundly beneficial impact on sleep too.

We now know, though, that for trauma, talking therapy is often not enough.

This is because, as we'll explore in depth later on, the effect of trauma is imprinted on a part of the brain that talking doesn't have much effect on. In fact, this part of the brain can *only be accessed through the body* and so it is essential to use the body (via breath and movement) to fully integrate the trauma.

And this 'bodywork' has to be done mindfully. This is because mindfulness has been shown to strengthen the connections to, and even increase, the density of the rational part of the brain, the prefrontal cortex, which gets knocked offline during traumatic experiences.[20]

This forms the basis of what has been called the 'bottom-up' body-based approach. The work of Dr Bessel van der Kolk, Dr Steven Porges' polyvagal theory, Dr Peter Levine's somatic experiencing, Dr Francine Shapiro's EMDR (Eye Movement Desensitization and Reprocessing), and EFT (Emotional Freedom Technique) Tapping all support this seemingly cutting-edge but actually ancient approach of integrating trauma.[21]

So, although talking therapy can be a great way to become aware of the trauma that we hold, and brilliant at helping us cognitively integrate the emotional baggage that trauma creates, the dysregulation of the brain that trauma leads to cannot simply be talked away. We must recalibrate the traumatized part of the brain through breath and bodywork and strengthen the connections to the rational, self-aware part of the brain through mindfulness practices.

The 'Mindfulness of Dream & Sleep' approach does exactly that.

~ Sleep Notes ~

If you're reading this book then you're most probably aspiring to integrate your stress or trauma so that you can sleep better, but what does 'integrate' actually mean? It comes from the Latin integrare, *'to make whole, to bring together, to unify'. The aim of the practices we'll learn in this book is to do just that: to make us feel whole so that we can sleep well again.*

A Gap in Our Knowledge

Most people know very little about how they sleep, and this lack of knowledge is not only harmful, but also disempowering. How can we even imagine making changes to our sleep when we know nothing about it?

It seems crazy that we leave the education system without learning anything about sleep. We know that we're going to be in this state for a third of our life and that one in 10 of us will have a major sleep disorder at some point,[22] and yet we don't think to teach our children about it?

In the next chapter we'll fill that gap in our knowledge by exploring not only how each stage of sleep works, but also how stress and trauma affect each one.

But just to highlight how little we as a society know about sleep, let's first explore a fascinating discovery about just how experimental our current sleeping habits are.

The Way We Used to Sleep

In 2011, when I was writing my first book, *Dreams of Awakening*, I came across a paper written by Roger Ekirch, Professor of History at Virginia Tech, titled: 'Sleep we have Lost: pre-industrial slumber in the British Isles'.[23] It was then that I first encountered the concept of the 'pre-industrial age sleep cycle'. It turns out that up until a couple of hundred years ago most people slept very differently from how we do today.

Nowadays, most industrial nations (with notable Hispanic exceptions) sleep monophasically, i.e. in one big chunk, but it turns out that before the early 1800s – and thus for a much longer period of human history – most people definitely got a healthy seven to nine hours each night, but fascinatingly it wasn't all in one go. Allowing for seasonal fluctuations, research shows that the first sleep period was from about 8–9 p.m. to midnight and the second from about 2 a.m. to dawn.

What was happening between midnight and 2 a.m.? People were doing stuff. They might go to a friend's place to smoke tobacco, they might pray (15th-century prayer manuals encourage it), have sex or even 'reflect on the dreams from their "first sleep"'.[24] Whatever they chose to do, one thing is for certain – most people were wide awake for a couple of hours right in the middle of the night.

In all probability, we slept in that way for thousands of years and many populations untouched by Western industrialization still have a similar sleeping pattern today.

~ *Sleep Notes* ~

A report from a 15th-century French missionary describes Brazilian tribes waking after a few hours of sleep to eat before returning for their 'second sleep', which lasted till dawn. With anthropological research finding more than 500 other cross-cultural references to this distinct 'two sleeps' pattern,[25] it can be assumed to have been an almost universal norm.

Coffee, Light Bulbs and Books

So what happened in the early 1800s to change the sleeping pattern we'd had for thousands of years? The Industrial Revolution happened, and with it the arrival of artificial light. Essentially, because the light afforded by candles was available only to the wealthiest families, most people went to sleep when the sun went down, but when gas–powered lighting arrived, soon followed by electric light, bedtimes were changed forever.

Add to this the arrival of coffee and, most fascinatingly of all, affordable books (and a new generation of people who knew how to read them), and suddenly people were staying up later, tanked up on caffeine, reading affordable novels by artificial light, and then waking early to work at gas-lit factories till way past sundown.

Professor Ekirch concluded that: 'This remarkably new form of monophasic sleep is a product not of the primeval past, but of forces grounded in the technology of artificial illumination and the shifting cultural attitudes toward sleep over the course of the Industrial Revolution.'[26]

Within just 50 years, these factors radically changed the way Brits slept and consequently affected the sleeping patterns of much of the world, 20 per cent of which was part of the British Empire.

Sleeping Guinea Pigs

Sadly, by the 1920s, the concept of a first and second sleep had receded entirely from our social consciousness, while over the same period a new concept was on the rise: insomnia. It is only in the early 20th century that insomnia 'as a distinct pathological and social label appears in Britain and the USA'[27] and an article in *The New York Times*[28] from 1900 bemoans this new-fangled malaise named 'insomnia'.

It wasn't just any insomnia, either. The most prevalent form was, and still is today, 'sleep maintenance insomnia' – a form in which people can get to sleep initially, but then wake up after a few hours and have trouble getting back to sleep. This condition first appears in medical literature in the late 1800s – exactly the same time that we stopped sleeping in two bouts.

Could this mean that there are thousands of misdiagnosed 'insomniacs' out there who are wide awake in the early hours not due to some dysfunction but simply a much more ancient (and possibly more natural) sleep cycle? Perhaps people who swear that they feel fine after four or five hours' sleep *really do* feel fine, but, regrettably, they aren't allowing themselves the second bout of sleep that is waiting for them in the wings.

Whatever the truth, it seems as though trying to sleep in one big chunk is still very much in the experimental stage and we are the unwitting guinea pigs.

The two main takeaways from this section on sleep history are:

- Our body may have a natural preference for segmented sleep and so it is totally okay to be awake in the middle in the night.

- If we can learn to relax into this night-time wakefulness, we may well find we can fall into the 'second sleep' that awaits us, as the normalization of this type of sleep is often all that is needed to allow people to relax into it.

CHAPTER 2

Knowledge Is Power

'The noblest pleasure is the joy of understanding.'
LEONARDO DA VINCI

As far as sleep is concerned, knowledge is power. Learning how sleep works and, crucially, how stress and trauma affect it empowers us to work with those effects. So the aim of this chapter is to demystify and destigmatize stress or trauma-affected sleep. By the end of it, I want you to know that however seemingly 'messed up' your sleep may seem, there is always a scientific explanation and always a chance of transformation.

If you've been traumatized in any way, whether by sexual assault, warzone experience, childhood neglect or abuse, an accident or losing someone close to you, your brain and body, and thus your sleep, will most probably be affected. That is totally normal.

Many people get used to living with these effects, but others quite naturally want them to stop and might go and see their local doctor. Russell Foster, Oxford University Professor of Neuroscience, says that most doctors know very little about sleep and although 'over 30 per cent of medical problems stem directly from sleep, sleep has been ignored in their medical training'.[1] My step-sister Holly, a newly qualified doctor, confirmed that she had just one two-hour module on sleep during her entire six-year medical training.

So, through no fault of their own, most doctors naturally tend to recommend what they know: either drugs, sleep hygiene tips[2] or both. These can be helpful for some people, but these approaches treat the symptoms and not the cause, which in the majority of cases is a nervous system riddled with stress.

The first things we can do to help reduce this stress are learn how sleep works and become aware of our own personal sleep cycle.

The Stages of Sleep

The Zen Buddhist master Thich Nhat Hanh says that awareness is like the sun: it transforms that which it shines upon. Awareness *in and of itself* is curative, and so simply being aware of how we are currently sleeping can help to transform our relationship to it.

Let's explore each of the four stages[3] of sleep in depth and learn exactly which techniques we can apply to mitigate the effects that stress or trauma might have on them.

Stage 1: The Hypnagogic State

This is the transitional state between wakefulness and sleep.

In the hypnagogic, our eyes are closed and we feel very drowsy, but we haven't actually fallen asleep yet, so we can still hear the sounds in the room and still feel our body in the bed. For many, the most recognizable aspect of this 'doorway into sleep' is the hypnagogic imagery: the dreamy hallucinations, both visual and auditory, that flash and fade in our mind's eye as we drift off. These psychedelic images are made up of memories of the day, mental preoccupations and displays of our subconscious mind.

While in the hypnagogic state, we might experience sudden bodily spasms, known as 'myoclonic jerks', which often become incorporated into hypnagogic 'micro-dreams', perhaps as stepping off a kerb or falling off a ledge. Some researchers believe this is an evolutionary throwback to when we used to sleep in trees – the jerk would help us maintain awareness of our sleeping place, so we didn't fall out of the tree. Others believe that it is the body's response to the steep drop in blood pressure that occurs when we pass through the hypnagogic unusually quickly. If we are sleep deprived we tend to hurtle through the hypnagogic as the body races towards the restorative sleep that lies beyond it; this sometimes makes the body respond with these little jolts. The main thing to know is that they are totally normal and simply an indication that you could do with a bit more sleep.

Neurologically, this stage of sleep is accompanied by alpha and theta brainwaves, which are associated with states of hypnosis and deep relaxation. This makes it a deeply suggestible and highly malleable state.

Although many people with problematic sleep find that the hypnagogic can be one of the most challenging sleep stages, it can be transformed into a state of deep potential if we can learn how to harness it.

How Might Stress or Trauma Affect Stage 1 Sleep?

A few years ago, I clashed heads in a kickboxing competition and broke my nose. That night, as soon as I entered the hypnogogic, I had flashbacks of that moment. As I lay there in bed with my eyes closed, I could see it so clearly, and I could even hear the crunch of bone. I would open my eyes and the flashback would stop, but as soon as I closed them again and entered the hypnagogic, they'd restart.

Trauma flashbacks (whether as minor as my head clash, or as serious as replays of a sexual assault, for example) may sometimes appear in the hypnagogic. As our brain switches from the linear, logical, left-brain dominance of the day to the intuitive, imaginal, right-brain dominance of the night, previously suppressed unconscious mental activity often pops up into conscious awareness in a shockingly uncensored fashion.

The way I explain it is through the medium of Whack-a-Mole.

Whack-a-Mole is a game that used to be found in fairgrounds and arcades all around the world. In it, you use a foam mallet to hit toy moles, which pop up at random and then sink back into their holes.

While we are awake, our mind does a similar thing to seemingly unwanted thoughts. Part of our mind, the egocentric preference system (a term coined by mindfulness expert Rob Nairn), is constantly trying to keep distressing or unpleasant thoughts out of our conscious awareness. All day every day it is playing Whack-a-Mole with our thoughts. When a distressing thought pops up, it says, 'Nope, I don't want to look at that!' and whacks it back down with the foam mallet of distraction, avoidance, denial or suppression. However, when we enter the hypnagogic state, the egocentric preference system falls asleep at its post. And when moles pop up, there's nothing to whack them back down again.

So, if you do find that you have flashbacks or intrusive traumatic thoughts in the hypnagogic state, know that it's a totally normal response to trauma and there are specific techniques that you can use to work with it.

Stress can affect the hypnagogic too. Racing thoughts, career worries, heartbroken rumination, fear of nightmares or simply an over-excited mind all serve to keep our stress response engaged and our relaxation response disengaged. Some of us can't even enter the hypnagogic, owing to hypervigilance, a mistrust of darkness or simply fear that one of those moles might pop up again.

However, for all the unpleasant ways in which the hypnagogic can be affected by stress or trauma, it is also one of the most malleable states of consciousness and one that responds quickly and effectively to certain practices.

Here are some of the practices that we can use to create peace in the hypnagogic. We'll explore them all in more detail later on, but for those of you who want to get stuck in straight away, check the list of exercises (*see p.xi*) to find their location in this book.

- The Nocturnal Journal

- Hypnagogic Mindfulness/Yoga Nidra

- Coherent Breathing/Breath-Body-Mind

- Circle of Protectors

- The 4,7,8 Breath

~ *Sleep Notes* ~

Without explanation or context, some of these practices probably sound a bit weird at first glance, but rest assured that we'll be exploring each one in detail later on. These lists of practices are designed to be used as a reference guide that you can use to create a tailored protocol of practices based on your specific sleep challenges.

Stage 2: Light Sleep

Following the half-awake/half-asleep hypnagogic state, we enter light sleep, where we experience the dissolution of external awareness and we black out.

As we enter light sleep, our heart rate starts to drop, our body temperature lowers, our eye movements stop and our brainwave activity slows down. Dreaming comes later in the sleep cycle, but if someone is woken from light sleep, they will often report thinking about something or exploring an idea. This is because light sleep plays a critical role in memory consolidation. It helps to consolidate declarative memories, such as factual information and new words or instructions, whereas dreaming sleep helps consolidate more complex and emotional memories.

Neurologically, light sleep is dominated by theta brainwaves, which are associated with flow states and meditation, interspersed with bursts of rapid, rhythmic brainwave activity known as sleep spindles.

Although it may not seem the most exciting sleep stage, we spend more time in light sleep than in any other stage and it makes up about 50 per cent of our total sleep time.

How Might Stress or Trauma Affect Stage 2 Sleep?

Compared to the other sleep stages, stress and trauma have no major *subjective* effects on this stage of sleep. However, they may affect our ability to enter it and, crucially, stay in it, so here are a couple of practices we can use to regulate and optimize this most prevalent of sleep states:

- Hypnagogic Mindfulness/Yoga Nidra

- Coherent Breathing/Breath–Body–Mind

Stage 3: Deep Sleep

As we fall further into slumber, our brain begins producing very low-frequency delta waves and we enter the deepest level of sleep.

In deep sleep, our brain is highly deactivated, and if we are woken from it, we'll commonly feel groggy and disorientated. It is a restorative sleep stage in which our heartbeat and breathing slow to their lowest rates and we quite literally detoxify our brain through an increased volume of cerebrospinal fluid,[4] which flushes out neurotoxins, including a protein called beta-amyloid that is linked to Alzheimer's disease. This process improves memory processing and consolidation, optimizes immune function and restores cell energy stores.[5]

As you can imagine, without deep sleep, our brain function is greatly impeded the next day.

Deep delta-wave sleep is also essential for general bodily repair, as it's the state in which HGH, human growth hormone, is released. This makes our cells regenerate and our hair, nails and muscles grow.

We get most of our deep sleep in the first four hours of our sleep cycle. This is why we can physically survive for quite a while on just four hours of sleep. But to thrive, rather than simply survive, it is essential to have the REM (rapid eye movement) dreaming sleep that follows it.

How Might Stress or Trauma Affect Stage 3 Sleep?

It's in deep sleep that parasomnias – things like sleepwalking, sleep talking and night terrors – might occur.

Sleepwalking is statistically pretty rare, but can be experienced as a result of high levels of stress, anxiety or illness, and can be genetically influenced as well.

It is not, as is often believed, the acting out of the physical movements corresponding to dream content, because we're not dreaming in deep sleep. How does it actually work? Although the motor systems are inhibited during all the stages of sleep (and totally inhibited during REM sleep), sometimes the movement systems in the sub-cortical brain tissue become activated during deep sleep, which is when this motor system inhibition is less active, leading to unconscious automatic movement.

Sleep talking, on the other hand, can happen in REM dreaming as well as deep sleep, and although it usually only affects about 5 per cent of adults, in populations working with trauma, this percentage is much higher.[6]

Night terrors, which are explored fully in Chapter 11, are often confused with nightmares, but in fact they aren't actually dreams at all, they're more like a form of night-time panic attack. They typically occur within the first four hours of sleep. Like sleepwalking or sleep talking, they are a totally natural response to stress or trauma, and thankfully there are lots of practices that can help to integrate the stress that triggers them, including:

• Hypnagogic Mindfulness/Yoga Nidra

• Coherent Breathing/Breath-Body-Mind

• Circle of Protectors

• 4-4-8 Alternate Nostril Breathing

• The 4,7,8 Breath

REM: Dreaming Sleep

After a long chunk of deep sleep, our brain switches from its most deactivated state to a state that is even more active than waking: REM sleep. That's when we dream.

We have our first dream period within about 90 minutes of falling asleep and although we do dream throughout the whole night, the majority of our dreaming is done in the last few hours of an eight-hour cycle.

Dreaming is an active sleep state – our brainwave activity, breathing and blood pressure all increase to near waking levels, while the actual process of dreaming requires so much neurological energy that it even burns calories.

Our body doesn't move, though – it becomes paralysed, so that we don't act out our dreams. A part of the brain called the pons sends a signal to the spinal cord to paralyse the major muscle groups.

As recently as a couple of decades ago the neuroscientific community was still unsure as to what the main purpose of dreaming actually was. But we now know that we dream in order to learn. 'REM sleep doesn't just hit the "save" button on memories, it actually hardwires them into the brain and then hits the "save" button.'[7]

Dreaming is also a way of updating our current memories in such a way that they aid our evolutionary survival by allowing our mind to replay and learn from past scenarios while also creatively rehearsing future scenarios. REM has been likened to a group psychotherapy session in which previously unconnected memories get to meet, connect and be integrated, while the members of the group share their concerns or worries about the future.

Sleep expert Professor Matthew Walker famously stated: 'We dream to remember and we dream to forget.'[8] We dream to *remember* the details of experiences of the day that might help to further our future wellbeing and to *forget* (let go of or integrate) the traumatic or painful emotional charge of past experiences.

Even though not everybody remembers their dreams, everybody does dream, every single night.[9] Dreaming is just as essential to our health as neurotoxin-removing deep sleep. In fact, when we're sleep-deprived, our brain actually prioritizes dreaming over the other three stages of sleep.

~ Sleep Notes ~

Just to clarify this point: dreaming is so beneficial and so beloved by the brain that if we miss a whole night's sleep, we'll get extra-long dream periods the following night. That's how important dreaming is to the brain.

How Might Stress or Trauma Affect REM Sleep?

Nightmares and anxiety dreams are the most obvious effects of stress and trauma on REM sleep. Nightmares are a totally normal response to stress and trauma, and Chapters 11 and 13 are dedicated to reframing them and learning techniques to integrate them.

As stated above, our body is paralysed while we dream, but sometimes, if we are having a highly emotional nightmare, 'motor breakthrough' can occur, when the paralysis mechanism of REM sleep is momentarily 'broken through'. This leads to sudden, usually singular body movements such as lashing out or kicking, which might be accompanied by shouting too.

Some people do occasionally thrash around in their sleep. If it only happens now and then, not to worry, but if you, or a loved one, regularly move around while asleep, and crucially if your movements match your dream content, it might be worth getting this checked out with a doctor, because it could be a sign of something called REM sleep behaviour disorder (RBD), which may require attention.[10]

There are a whole host of practices that we can use to integrate nightmares and anxiety dreams, such as:

- Coherent Breathing/Breath-Body-Mind

- Circle of Protectors

- The 4,7,8 Breath

- 4-4-8 Alternate Nostril Breathing

- Nightmare Rescripting

- Lucid Dreaming

The Hypnopompic State

The final sleep stage is more of a transitional state than a sleep stage proper. It's the state of mind between sleep and wakefulness, the hypnopompic state. In this state, our eyes are still closed, but we can hear the sounds in the room and we are no longer asleep or dreaming, but not quite awake either.

Just as the hypnagogic is the doorway into sleep, the hypnopompic is the doorway out. It contains much less mental imagery than the hypnagogic, though, and because we are partially awake but not yet fully conscious, it's often experienced as a kind of broad panoramic awareness.

There is often an extended hypnopompic period that occurs naturally after the first three 90-minute sleep cycles. Some of us will wake up at this point (ever noticed how you might wake up spontaneously about four to five hours after going to sleep?), while others may simply come to rest in the semi-awake state of the hypnopompic.

The hypnopompic is a very fresh state of mind, enlivened by the rejuvenation of the sleep that has preceded it. This gives it a kind of magnified clarity that explains why we often have inspired insights upon awakening.

How Might Stress or Trauma Affect the Hypnopompic State?

Owing to its similarity with the hypnagogic state and the fact that the egocentric preference system is usually still booting up, whatever we have been suppressing during our waking hours may pop up into the hypnopompic state too. The enhanced clarity we experience may shine a light into the dark corners of our mind, revealing hidden fears as well as inspired insights.

Accordingly, if we are working with stress or trauma, this particular stage of our sleep cycle may often unwittingly illuminate whatever heartbreak, tragedy or stressful life event we have been trying to avoid thinking about. This is sometimes referred to as 'the 4 a.m. demons', a state of anxiety or mental rumination that usually occurs after about four to five hours of sleep. It often shocks us awake and leaves us lying there, confronted by the thoughts we have been trying to avoid.

The hypnopompic also plays host to sleep paralysis, an often hallucinatory experience in which we wake from sleep feeling totally paralysed, with images superimposed over our normal field of vision. This can be a terrifying experience, but the terror is mostly rooted in the mystery of the situation. In Chapter 11 we explore sleep paralysis in depth.

Sleep paralysis and the 4 a.m. demons are totally natural responses to both trauma and the stresses of everyday life. They are both relatively common and we can work with them through practices such as:

- The Nocturnal Journal and 'worry writing'

- Hypnagogic Mindfulness/Yoga Nidra

- Coherent Breathing/Breath-Body-Mind

- Hypnopompic Mindfulness

The Journey through Sleep

Sleep is a cyclical journey that progresses from hypnagogic drowsiness through light sleep, down into the depths of deep sleep and then up into the realm of dreaming every 90 minutes or so, multiple times throughout the night. With each of these cycles we spend increasingly more time in REM dreaming and increasingly less time in deep sleep. So the first few hours are mainly deep sleep with short dream periods and then, once we have our deep sleep under our belt, we move into longer REM periods.

It's worth mentioning that most of us have brief awakenings throughout the night, often at the end of each 90-minute cycle, but because we ordinarily don't have any memory of them, we think we've slept constantly.

People with problematic sleep, however, tend to grasp at these micro-awakenings and panic, because of their hyper-conscious fear of not being able to sleep when they should be asleep. This reaction causes their brain to awaken even further and stress hormones to be released, and so perpetuates the cycle.

In 13 years of teaching workshops on sleep and dreams, I have yet to meet anyone who sleeps in a perfect four-stage 90-minute sleep cycle, so please use the information in this chapter simply as a rough framework for exploring how *you* sleep. Your aim here is to empower yourself with knowledge, not to get hung up on the fact that you don't sleep in exactly the same way as others.

➤ Field-Tested Feedback

A woman who had been receiving treatment for cancer at the time of doing the 'Mindfulness of Dream & Sleep' course said, 'All the sleep stages stuff and learning how stress can affect them was really helpful. It helped me to understand that being awake in the middle of the night is okay and so I no longer find it distressing. If I do wake up now, I can just drift back to sleep. I sleep more deeply now too and I feel less anxious during the day.'

Another participant said, 'It really helped me understand why I am having issues with my sleep, so I feel a lot less anxious about it now. It helped me to be curious rather than fearful about going to sleep.'

•••

The Indian philosopher Krishnamurti once said, 'The seeing is the doing,' to encapsulate his belief that just by being aware of something, we can change it for the better. So too with our sleep: simply by learning about how it works, we can radically transform our relationship to it.

This leads us to our first technique: keeping a Nocturnal Journal.

CHAPTER 3

Documenting Sleep: The Nocturnal Journal

'Man is a genius when he is dreaming.'
AKIRA KUROSAWA, FILM-MAKER

People with a stressful or traumatized relationship to sleep are often unwilling to take a good look at it, and understandably so: sleep is a state they associate with fear or failure, or even with the trauma itself. However, as paradoxical as it may seem, if we become more aware of our sleep experience, the warm gaze of our fascination might start to melt the icy relationship we have with it.[1]

The awareness of one type of sleep in particular plays a vital role in both the integration of trauma and our everyday mental health: dreaming.

Dream Awareness for Mental Health

Research shows that only about 2 per cent of our dreams are a straight replay of our daily life[2] and that the rest are a reflection of the emotional themes and concerns of our daily life.[3] Dreams reveal the internal environment of our psyche, what Virginia Woolf once described as the 'submerged truth' of who we are, and so by becoming aware of our dreams, we become aware of that truth.

In fact, new research suggests that even when we aren't aware of it, that truth is still there. Neuroscientists at the University of California, Berkeley, believe that being able to remember a dream hours or even days after it happened proves that the memory of our dreams is stored within us, even if we can't remember our dreams when we first wake up.[4] And so the psychological charge of those dreams can have a huge impact on our waking state at a subconscious level.

Shockingly, this means that every time we wake from a dream that we don't remember, the underlying emotional tone of that dream, whether uplifting or depressing, will be having an effect on our waking life. Essentially, our unremembered dreams are affecting our waking-state wellbeing.

Could it be that millions of people are waking up each morning feeling depressed or inexplicably on edge, due to the psychological charge of an anxiety dream they don't recall? This is one of the best arguments I have ever come across for recalling and documenting our dreams every day, because the simple act of remembering them (and even better writing them down or talking about them) helps to discharge this emotional energy and prevent it from negatively impacting our day.

A New View of Anxiety Dreams

You know those dreams where you're at the train station and can't find the right platform or you're at the airport and can't find your passport? Although you may wake from them feeling anxious, they might not be such a bad thing. In the nights preceding an important event, like a holiday or an exam, our brain uses REM sleep to run through worst-case scenarios so that we're better prepared to face those scenarios, should they occur in the waking state. By presenting us with those scenarios, our brain is actually trying to help us. What's the first thing you do after a pre-holiday 'lost passport' dream? Locate your passport. Anxiety dreams are not designed to stress you out but rather to prevent stressful events coming to pass by making you better equipped to avoid them.

THE SCIENCE OF ANXIETY DREAMS

There is solid science behind anxiety dreams. A 2014 study[5] headed by Isabelle Arnulf, president of the French Society for Sleep Research and Sleep Medicine, collected the dreams of hundreds of students from the Sorbonne medical school doing their final exams. The Sorbonne finals are extremely competitive – fewer than 10 per cent of students make the grade – so they naturally give rise to high levels of anxiety.

Many of the students had anxiety dreams the night before their final exam or in the nights leading up to it. Some dreamed of being late because of train delays, others of not being able to find the exam hall, and one student even dreamed that they were given a slice of bread instead of the exam paper.

Fascinatingly, the study found that those who had the anxiety dreams did significantly better in the exam than the students who did not. The researcher commented, 'Whatever happened in their brain as they dreamed the night before, it gave a cognitive gain compared with the other students.'[6]

In fact, the top five marks went to students who had had an anxiety dream the night before the final exam. One of the Sorbonne students actually dreamed that she was revising, but didn't know an important detail about the spinal cord. She then woke up from the dream, looked up the detail in question and memorized it. The next day a question about that very same detail came up in the exam paper! Spooky, eh?

So it seems that the ebb and flow of the dreaming mind affects the tides of our conscious experience, but if we can train ourselves to remember our dreams and to discharge the memories by writing them down or saying them out loud, we can free ourselves from whatever unconscious effect they are having on our daily life.

Our first tool in what will eventually be a 21-piece toolbox is a great way to do exactly that.

Exercise: The Nocturnal Journal

In this exercise you'll be taking note, in a 'Nocturnal Journal', of how you've slept, how much sleep you're getting and your mental state on awakening. The main reason for doing this is initially to get a baseline for how you are sleeping now, so you can chart how it changes over the next few weeks.

You should also make a note of your dreams, if possible. Paradoxical insomnia, the belief that you have lain awake all night when actually you've been asleep, can be combatted by being aware of your dreams, because if you can remember a dream then you have *proof* that you most probably had a big chunk of deep sleep before it. This can have a really beneficial psychological impact.

For now, your main focus is on getting a solid baseline for how you're sleeping, but later on you'll start to focus more on remembering your dreams as a way of preparing the ground for the lucid dreaming practices of Part V.

How does keeping a Nocturnal Journal actually work?

It's just like keeping a daytime journal, but rather than focusing on the content of your day, you focus on the content of your night. Each morning you write, draw or somehow note down a general overview of your nocturnal experience. This will be divided in two main parts: sleep and dreams.

The sleep part will take note of:

~ the time you went to bed and woke up

~ the process of falling asleep

~ any sleep stages that you were aware of

~ how many hours of sleep you had

~ any daytime factors that may have impacted your sleep

~ how you felt on awakening

And the dream part will take note of:

~ any dreams you can remember

~ the main themes and emotional tone of them

~ how you felt about them upon awakening

If you don't usually remember you dreams, it's helpful to set a strong intention to recall them before bed.

If you can, for a few minutes as you're falling asleep, recite over and over in your mind: *Tonight, I remember my dreams. I have excellent dream recall.*

Most people will be able to recall at least part of their dreams without too much difficulty after just a couple of nights of doing this, even if they haven't recalled a dream in years. For more tips on how to recall your dreams see Chapter 15.

Every time you make an entry in your Nocturnal Journal, you are creating and reinforcing the habit of viewing your sleep and dreams as valuable. This creates a bi-directional positive feedback loop in which your conscious mind will become more aware of how you're sleeping (because of your conscious intention to do so) and your unconscious mind will start to present you with more memorable dreams (because it now knows that you want to remember them).

I know that may sounds a bit woo-woo, but it's true: over 80 per cent of the six-week 'Mindfulness of Dream & Sleep' course participants found that they became more aware of both their sleep cycle and their dreams within a few weeks simply by setting their intention to do so and by keeping a Nocturnal Journal.[7]

—————————————————

Here is an example of a Nocturnal Journal entry:

12 August 2020

Bed at 11 p.m., but lights out at 11.30 p.m. after scrolling social media on my phone for 30 minutes.

Took ages to fall asleep (maybe all the Instagram scrolling?) and was in the hypnagogic for what felt like forever, but eventually fell asleep.

Set a strong intention to remember my dreams as I was falling asleep, though.

Woke a few hours later to pee and remembered a long dream about being at work but the office looked like my primary school. My brother was there too, but he looked like that French kid from primary school. I was searching for something, but I can't remember what exactly. It felt a bit ominous, but I didn't seem to be acting as if I was afraid at all.

Struggled to get back to sleep afterwards and felt wide awake, so I read a book for a bit, did some slow breathing and eventually got back to sleep.

Alarm went off at 7 a.m., but I hit the snooze and just rested in the hypnopompic for a bit before slipping back into sleep. Woke at 7.30 and knew I had been dreaming, but can't remember what.

Felt pretty good once I got out of bed. Much better than yesterday, anyway.

Overall Sleep

Probably about six or seven hours I think, but I was in bed for eight.

Pre-Sleep Factors

Worried about not getting enough sleep, so scrolled Instagram to try to forget about it.

Blue light from phone screen and overstimulation from the content I was reading = took ages to fall asleep.

Daytime Factors

Quite stressed at work (maybe that explains the office dream?)

Did 20 minutes of breathwork practice during the day (pretty sure that's why I didn't freak out when I was awake in the middle of the night).

Was reading about the benefits of hypnopompic state a few days ago (gave me confidence to rest there after hitting snooze button).

Top Tips for Nocturnal Journals

- When you wake up in the morning, recall and document your sleep and dream experience straight away, or else you might forget it.

- You don't need to record every tiny detail, but you'll be surprised how much you can write up in just five minutes or so.

- Don't jump out of bed as soon as you wake up, just lie there for a moment and see if you can catch the feeling or tone of a particular emotion in your body. This may help to unlock the memory of your dreams.

- If you're using your smartphone for your Nocturnal Journal, rather than a pen and notebook (either method is fine), make sure that the screen brightness is turned right down and that it is in airplane mode to avoid disturbances and distractions.

- Avoid clockwatching. Adding up your sleep hours in the middle of the night will activate the left-hemisphere (logical) brain areas that you need to deactivate in order to get to sleep. Be mildly interested yet wholly unconcerned about the times you wake up in the middle of the night.

- If you have a sleep-tracker device, feel free to use it, but don't take the data too seriously. Any that track movement via an accelerometer (which include the vast majority) are particularly untrustworthy, as every time your partner moves or the cat jumps on the bed it may register a false wake-up or change of sleep state.

~ Sleep Notes ~

Sleep trackers can often cause anxiety and sometimes even make us feel worse. On many occasions people have told me that they thought they had had a great night's sleep until they checked their sleep tracker and it told them they hadn't! If a tracker helps you feel more confident about your sleep, then feel free to keep using it, but it's even better to become your own sleep tracker by keeping a Nocturnal Journal and by trusting how you feel in the morning, not how your sleep tracker says you should feel.

Worry Writing

Feel free to use some of the pages in your Nocturnal Journal for 'worry writing' too. If you find that you can't get to sleep because your mind is racing, then writing down all of the anxious thoughts or worries that are keeping you awake can be a great way to get to sleep.

The anxious thoughts, just like us, want to be seen and heard, so writing them down not only helps to do this but it also helps to download and discharge the emotional energy of those thoughts.

Be sure to remind yourself that the middle of the night isn't the best time to problem-solve, though, and if you can, schedule a time the next day to address the things that are worrying you. Setting the intention to address a certain problem at a specific date or time in the future is a very effective way of allowing the brain to put that worry aside.

This particular aspect of the technique can be really helpful for some people.

➤ Field-Tested Feedback

After a week of keeping his Nocturnal Journal, my friend Tony, who runs the Forward Assist veterans' charity, emailed to say, 'You're right, Charlie... knowledge is power. Slept for five-and-a-half hours straight on day three of keeping my sleep journal. That's unheard of. And it added an extra 30 mins to my sleep time too!'

On the first night of the first Veterans' Mindfulness Retreat that I ever taught on, I gave an opening session based on what we've learned in this book so far. The next morning, we had a group sharing of our Nocturnal Journals in which one of the veterans said, with wet, joyful eyes, 'I did it! I slept through… the whole night! I still woke early with the demons, but I knew it was okay. It was even about four hours after I went down, too, like he said. I didn't panic and just went back to sleep!'

Then in the tea break that followed, another veteran, a gunner named Matt who'd served in the Falklands War, told me quietly: 'It's good, this is. Just learning how it all works makes it okay.'

And then, just before he walked away, he said something so poetic that it's been imprinted on my memory ever since: 'It's like we've got a new circle. We used to have a circle of despair, but now we've got a circle of hope.'

Part I Checklist ✓

✓ Aim to understand how all of the various sleep stages work and how stress and trauma can affect each one.

✓ Allow yourself to become fascinated by your personal sleep cycle.

✓ Start keeping a Nocturnal Journal every day, if possible.

✓ Notice how your sleep changes in response to you offering it your attention.

✓ Go and get yourself a pillow – you'll need it for Part II.

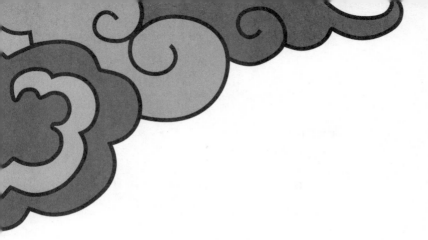

PART II

REST AND RELAX

*'The most valuable thing we can do
for the psyche is to let it rest.'*

MAY SARTON, POET

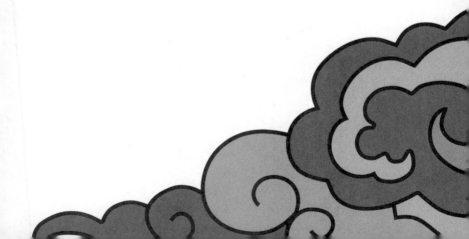

Now that we've empowered ourselves with the knowledge of how sleep works and started to become interested in how we sleep, we'll turn our attention to sleep's favourite cousin: rest.

Rest is the bridge that leads to sleep, so we must learn how to rest well if we are to learn how to sleep well.

In this section we'll learn some of the most effective techniques available for relaxing deeply and resting soundly.

But first we need to learn about what stops us from relaxing into rest: stress.

CHAPTER 4

Stressed–Out Sleep

'Many things, such as loving and going to sleep...
are done worst when we try hardest to do them.'
C.S. LEWIS

The man who first taught me about mindfulness and sleep, meditation teacher Rob Nairn, once told me, 'Insomnia is the process of trying to fall asleep.'

Falling asleep isn't something you can *try* to do. In fact, sleep is, in many ways, the culmination of not doing anything at all. It is an automatic biological process that will occur naturally in the absence of stressors that prevent it from occurring.

Most of the sleep hygiene approaches to troubled sleep largely ignore these internal biological stressors, and focus instead on external obstacles such as blue-frequency light and caffeine intake. The core of the approach seems to be: remove the external obstacles to sleep in order to create conditions that make it easier to fall asleep.

Some of these sleep hygiene hacks can be quite helpful, so I've listed a few of the best ones in the appendix. They include things like accessing rest before trying to access sleep and keeping your bedroom as cool, dark and sleep-friendly as possible.

Sleep hygiene tips aren't long-term solutions, though, and can often become further obstacles to sleep as we stress ourselves out over creating the perfect external conditions. Author of *The Sleep Book* Dr Guy Meadows sums this up perfectly: 'They often become one of many props that contribute to the general loss of trust in our own ability to sleep.'[1]

Sleep hygiene is a bit like dental hygiene – it can certainly help prevent problems from occurring, but once you have a problem, something more fundamental is required.

We must focus on changing the *internal environment* of our body rather than simply the external environment of our bedroom if we want a long-term solution to sleeplessness.

We can be using all the blue-light-filtering technology in the world, but unless we filter out the biological stressors that are preventing sleep from occurring, we may well be stuck staring at the ceiling till dawn.

Three of the most prominent of these biological stressors are:

- stress (including anxiety and worry)

- inflammation (the underlying symptom of almost all illness)

- trauma (both psychological and physical)

Later on we will explore each one in depth, but before that we need to explore the bodily system that they all affect: the autonomic nervous system (ANS).

The Gatekeeper of Sleep

The autonomic nervous system (ANS) is the part of the nervous system that controls any bodily functions that aren't consciously directed. Which turns out to be the vast majority of them. Things like breathing, heart rate, hormone release, brain function, immune response, digestion and sleep.

Because over 90 per cent per cent of our bodily functions are controlled by our ANS, if *it* is working well, *we* are working well. In fact, if we can get our ANS in balance, we won't need to try to sleep, as sleep will happen naturally.

The ANS is made up of two parts: the sympathetic and the parasympathetic.

The Sympathetic Nervous System

Often called the 'fight or flight' response, the sympathetic nervous system uses adrenaline to activate our ability to fight or flee in the face of perceived dangers and provides our body with a burst of energy for those responses. It's a bit like the accelerator pedal in a car: it leads to speed and action. It makes our heart beat faster, pulse rate and blood pressure go up and breathing rate increase, all within a split-second of our brain registering the threat.

The 'fight of flight' system creates hormonal changes too: our adrenal glands start pumping adrenaline into our bloodstream, closely followed by cortisol. These 'stress hormones' put our body into a state of high alert. When the threat has passed, our body releases other hormones to help our muscles relax and our ANS returns to an equilibrium. In theory, anyway.

However, the fast-paced Westernized lifestyle that most of us live nowadays creates an internal environment dominated by stress, which in turn leads to an over-activation of the sympathetic 'fight or flight' system. This means that most of us spend the majority of our life in a state of low-level 'fight or flight' activation, in which our body is constantly prepared for a threat that never comes.

In his book *The New Science of Breath*, Stephen Elliott describes this state as 'chronic sympathetic dominance'.[2] It means that our brain pumps out way more stress hormones than needed, which leads to a major imbalance in the ANS. This process releases more free radicals and increases inflammation,[3] while leading to high blood pressure, digestive problems, anxiety and the risk of heart attacks and strokes (due to the artery-clogging deposits that stress hormones create).

It also leads to premature ageing, because it's like pressing the accelerator pedal in our car when we're parked up with the handbrake on. It wears out the engine and ruins the car.

And of course, all this is terrible for sleep as well, because sympathetic activation creates the production of cortisol: the alertness hormone. For sleep to occur, we need to switch off the 'fight or flight' system and activate the other branch of the ANS: the parasympathetic system.

But before we explore the parasympathetic system, it's worth noting that there are third and fourth options linked to the 'fight or flight' response: freeze and fawn.

Freezing, also called reactive immobility or attentive immobility, can be seen as 'fight or flight' on hold. We can't run away or fight, so instead we become immobile. Just like 'fight or flight', the freeze response isn't a conscious decision. It's an automatic reaction, so we can't control it.

There are some interesting new theories positing that some types of depression might actually be a manifestation of the freeze response. In some cases, the constant overactivity of the 'fight or flight' system eventually blows the fuse and we enter into the freeze state, which is often misdiagnosed as depression. If this is correct, it would mean that depression, just like trauma, is a nervous system condition and so talk therapy and/or drugs might not be the best approach for it either.

The fawn response (first coined by Pete Walker in his brilliant book *Complex PTSD: From Surviving to Thriving*) is triggered when we respond to danger by trying to placate the threat or attacker by being helpful or pleasing towards them. Essentially, we seek safety by attempting to diffuse the threat by appeasing the attacker. Fawning (just like fight, flight and freeze) is an automatic response to threat, so we are no more able to prevent it than the other three.

The Parasympathetic Nervous System

The parasympathetic 'rest and digest' system is very different: it's like the brake pedal in a car. It calms down our body and mind, allowing us to relax and revive.

When the parasympathetic system is engaged, our heart rate drops, our breathing slows down and our cells begin to repair themselves. Mentally, we feel relaxed, as our mind calms down, while on a physical level, inflammation is reduced, energy reserves are restored[4] and our digestive system switches on, hence 'rest and digest'.

Parasympathetic activation is just as linked to our survival as 'fight or flight'. Both to have sex and eat we need it to be activated. The reason why men struggle to get an erection and women struggle to have an orgasm if they are anxious is again because stress and anxiety prevent the activation of the parasympathetic system. Similarly, the reason we often lose our appetite when we're grief-stricken is that the stress of grief activates 'fight or flight' and deactivates 'rest and digest', and with it the desire to eat.

Conversely, although still logically, some people feel the desire to eat more when grieving (comfort eating). Trauma specialist Dr Heather Sequeira told me, 'This is because high carb intake can facilitate the uptake of tryptophan, which temporarily decreases levels of stress and arousal. Unfortunately, eating simple carbs also increases levels of inflammation in the body, which then creates more stress, so it's a delicate and difficult issue for many.'[5]

Whereas the 'fight or flight' system switches on very quickly (but takes time to switch off), the 'rest and digest' system switches on relatively slowly. In fact, it often needs to be consciously activated by doing relaxing things like lying down or slowing our breathing or simply creating conditions that make us feel both psychologically and physically safe and relaxed.

How does all this relate to sleep?

As you might imagine, sleep requires a state of *parasympathetic activation*.

Sleep and the ANS

To fall asleep and stay asleep we need to balance the ANS by turning off 'fight or flight' and turning on 'rest and digest'. As Dr Alan Christianson says, cortisol is our 'built-in coffee pot',[6] so although it's great for waking us up, until our brain stops pumping it out, we'll be far too alert to sleep.

Most of the techniques in this book are specifically designed to reduce the levels of those stress hormones and allow us to activate the parasympathetic system before sleep. In fact, two of them, Yoga Nidra and Coherent Breathing, have been scientifically proven to be two of the most effective techniques for balancing the ANS, thus leading to improved sleep.

Now that we know how the ANS works, let's get back to the three primary biological stressors that dysregulate it.

Stress, Inflammation and Trauma

Stress, inflammation and trauma all feed off and exacerbate one another. In many ways, they are all both symptomatic and causal of one another.

They all lead to 'fight or flight' over-activation and a dysregulated ANS. This creates more inflammation, which leads to more stress response, and so the vicious circle continues. All this is bad news not only for our sleep, but for our all-round health too.

The good news is that if we can learn how to reduce the levels of stress and inflammation in our body, while integrating the effects of trauma on our brain, we can begin to sleep and live soundly again.

Stress

We all know what it feels like to be stressed – the mental or physical feeling of tension or pressure that is the opposite of feeling relaxed. Stress can be medically defined as the body's reaction to 'any change that requires an adjustment or response'.[7] All change, even pleasant change like a promotion or the birth of a child, creates a level of stress, and the human body is designed to cope with it.

In fact, low levels of intermittent stress are actually good for us. There is a phenomenon called stress immunization that demonstrates that exposure to a moderate level of stress from childhood onwards can immunize us against stress overload in later life.[8]

So, stress isn't bad, but chronic stress and the *sympathetic dominance* that it leads to are.

Inflammation

Sleep expert Professor Rubin Naiman believes that inflammation is the most overlooked issue in disturbed sleep. Inflammation is a biological defence mechanism in which the immune system recognizes damaged cells and begins the healing process by triggering bodily responses such as scabbing, swelling and bruising. These allow our wounds and damaged tissues to heal.

So, just like stress, intermittent bouts of inflammation are needed to protect our health, but when inflammation persists when it is not needed, it can become harmful. Chronic inflammation underlies most major illnesses, from heart disease to rheumatoid arthritis to depression, anxiety and even PTSD. A 2020 a metanalysis of 50 medical papers found direct links between inflammation and PTSD, both as a contributing factor and a symptom.[9]

Inflammation also underlies chronic sleeplessness. Not only does it activate the 'fight or flight' system, which prevents sleep, but it also results in a slight but clinically significant increase in body temperature,[10] which may, owing to sleep being closely linked to a decrease in body temperature, prevent us from falling asleep at all.

The two main ways to reduce chronic inflammation are by activating the parasympathetic system, through its connection to the vagal nerve network, and by adjusting our diet.

Avoiding inflammatory foods, such as refined carbs, fried foods, processed and red meat and of course sugar, while eating more anti-inflammatory foods, such as fish, nuts, berries, vegetables and olive oil among others, is one of the most direct ways to improve both your sleep and your general health.

A 2016 study in the *Journal of Clinical Sleep Medicine* found that a diet high in inflammatory sugar and carbs but low in fibre led to less deep sleep and more night-time awakenings[11] and a Canadian medical study found that for those who consumed fewer than three sources of fruit and vegetables daily, there were at least 24 per cent higher odds of anxiety disorder diagnosis,[12] and the troubled sleep caused by it.

Well-known anti-inflammatory supplements such as vitamin D, zinc, turmeric and omega oils are all great too, but if you want to really tap into the power of nature, check out Rhodiola rosea, astaxanthin, ashwagandha and the amazing Himalayan plant-based resin shilajit. Those four all come highly recommended for reducing inflammation and aiding sleep, have a huge range of other benefits and are safe for most people, including those working with trauma.

Also, sleep itself is a potent anti-inflammatory, so just as reducing inflammation will improve our sleep, improving our sleep will reduce inflammation.

Trauma

We will explore trauma and PTSD in depth later, when we have some more practical tools to navigate the exploration, but for now let's touch on the basics.

Psychologically speaking, trauma is the effect of any stressful experience that overwhelms a person's ability to cope and to integrate their response to that stressful experience.

Biologically, it creates a dysregulation of the autonomic nervous system that makes the 'fight or flight' system more easily activated and the 'rest and digest' response less easily activated. Many of the symptoms of trauma – anxiety, depression, hypervigilance, sleeplessness – are caused not so much by the trauma itself, but more by the dysregulation of the ANS that the trauma creates.

It is an individual's *subjective experience* that determines whether an event is traumatic. Some people may be traumatized by a warzone experience, others by social media bullying. Just as a broken heart can be worse than a death for some, and a pet dying can be worse than losing a human family member for others, trauma is highly personal. If an event has such a strong impact on you that you are overwhelmed by the stressful effects and unable to integrate them, then that absolutely counts as trauma, so please don't feel that your trauma isn't 'enough'.

In summary, troubled sleep is caused primarily by a dysregulated ANS, which in turn is caused by the effects of stress, inflammation and trauma on the body.

Professor Chris Idzikowski, asleep disorder specialist, agrees: 'Insomnia is caused by hyperarousal, a state in which a person's brain is simply too activated to sleep.'[13]

In order to sleep well, we need to be able to dial down the hyperarousal of the 'fight or flight' system and switch on the 'rest and digest' system.

One of the easiest ways to do that is with the deeply relaxing practices of hypnagogic mindfulness and Yoga Nidra.

CHAPTER 5

Hypnagogic Mindfulness

'The hypnagogic state is considered by many to be a genius state, without boundaries or any limitations.'

DR BRIAN WEISS, BESTSELLING AUTHOR OF
MANY LIVES, MANY MASTERS

It is the graveyard shift at the Veterans' Mindfulness Retreat in Scotland.[1] As the participants make their final adjustments to their lying-down meditation areas, I am battling against both the post-lunch carb drop and the good-natured banter that you come to expect from a group of ex-military.

'Don't you start snoring again, Tommy!'

'It's not the snoring you need to worry about, pal, it's Keith's farting!'

'I do *not* fart!'

The group of 25 is made up of military veterans, serving military personnel and veterans' family members. They are spaced out evenly, each lying on a yoga mat or blanket with a pillow under their head. With smiles on their faces, they get ready for…

'Nap time!'

'It's not a nap! He said that last time! Listen up, will ya?'

'I was trying, but I couldn't hear him over your snoring!'

When you work with veterans, you need to be ready for the banter; it's a vital part of the bonding process and forms a big part of the 'invisible therapy' that happens at these retreats.

I begin my introduction: 'This technique is about learning to rest on the drowsy boundary of sleep without actually falling asleep. It's called hypnagogic mindfulness. As you know, the hypnagogic state is the doorway that leads into sleep. And mindfulness is the faculty of mind that *knows what's happening as it's happening*. So, this practice is about being mindfully aware within the state just before sleep. Awareness is the crucial factor here. It's awareness that prevents us from falling asleep. Remember, this is not nap time…'

'See, I told ya!'

'This is deep relaxation time, so set a strong intention to maintain mindful awareness throughout. If you do fall asleep, that's totally fine, and maybe it's what your body needs, but if you start snoring, then…'

'That's you, eh, Tommy!'

'...then you will hear the Tibetan singing bowl. If you do hear it, just become aware of your breathing and carry on. There's no shame in snoring, no shame in falling asleep. All I ask is that you explore the possibility of staying aware throughout.'

'Aye, fair enough, pal.'

And with that ultimate Scottish seal of approval, they settle down and begin the practice.

The Doorway into Sleep

Hypnagogic mindfulness is about learning to relax deeply on the doorway into sleep. This kind of practice has been shown to directly decrease sympathetic 'fight or flight' activity while increasing parasympathetic 'rest and digest' function and vagal tone activation. It helps our body to get into the habit of being more relaxed at all times.

By intentionally accessing the doorway into sleep, we are helping our body start to remember that it can be accessed and that sleep can occur totally naturally. The reason that this practice is so good for insomniacs is that if we can consciously learn the route to sleep in the daytime, then we can follow that route again at night-time. I know it seems paradoxical, but by learning how *not* to fall asleep, we will actually train our body to remember *how* to fall asleep.

Yoga Nidra

One of the most popular forms of hypnagogic mindfulness is an ancient practice called Yoga Nidra.

When we hear the word 'yoga', we usually think of the movement sequences and bodily postures that form the most common type of yoga practised in the West. But the Sanskrit word *yoga* actually means 'union' and has nothing to do with movement sequences as such.

Nidra is another Sanskrit word, meaning 'sleep', so Yoga Nidra can be translated as 'sleep union' or 'the sleep that is unified'. Unified with what? With awareness.

As part of the Lucid Dreaming Summit that I organized with the Awake Academy online platform during the 2020 lockdown, I interviewed my friend and Yoga Nidra expert Uma Dinsmore-Tuli, PhD, on her specialist subject.

Uma explained that Yoga Nidra is 'a meditation on the moment of falling asleep. You meditate on the experience of being in the hypnagogic state. You lie down and either guide yourself into that state or in most cases you listen to a guided audio track. Some of these contain complex visualizations with set scripts, but actually neither of those are necessary. All that is necessary for Nidra is meditation on the moment of falling asleep.'[2]

The Benefits of Yoga Nidra

Yoga Nidra is really good for you. As Uma explained, 'It functions equally as a meditative practice and a therapeutic tool. Yoga Nidra can promote deep healing and a very profound state of rest at all levels – physical, mental, emotional and spiritual. It can be used to relieve insomnia, anxiety, depression, panic attacks and other stress-related problems. It's great for chronic pain management too.'

She told me about an eight-week Yoga Nidra study with Vietnam veterans who were experiencing intrusive memories and trauma flashbacks. During and after the course, they reported reduced levels of rage, anxiety and reactivity and increased feelings of relaxation, peace, self-awareness and self-efficacy.

Uma quoted the PTSD UK founder Jacqui Suttie, who said, 'Yoga Nidra can be considered a highly effective practice for reducing stress and PTSD symptoms.'

I asked her if there were any drawbacks or groups of people who shouldn't do Yoga Nidra and she replied, 'No, that's the best part – everyone can do it and it seems to help a huge range of ailments.'

THE SCIENCE OF YOGA NIDRA

Studies have shown that practising Yoga Nidra in the daytime leads to 'significant improvement in sleep-quality due to it creating an increased parasympathetic drive at night'.[3]

Studies on iRest, a form of Yoga Nidra currently offered in military hospitals across the USA, have consistently shown that it can help to 'increase ability to handle PTSD, pain and stress' while also helping to 'decrease body tension, improve quality of sleep [and] the ability to handle intrusive thoughts and to manage stress'.[4]

A 2018 study exploring the effects of Yoga Nidra on stressed-out university professors found significant improvement in positive wellbeing, general health and vitality in those who practised it. When they looked at the brains of the stressed profs, they found that Yoga Nidra practice led to 'an integrated response by the hypothalamus, resulting in decreased sympathetic and increased parasympathetic relaxation'.[5]

This confirms an earlier neurobiological study that found that Yoga Nidra 'decreases activity in regions involved in emotional processing and motor planning, which leads to an increase in both physical and mental relaxation while reducing anxiety levels'.

More Relaxing than Sitting

Practices like Yoga Nidra are often even better for creating deep relaxation than sitting meditation practices.[6] This is partly because we're lying down and partly because it's not actually necessary to concentrate as much. Yoga Nidra is usually guided by an audio track, so all we need to do is to follow the instructions, maintain awareness and ideally not fall asleep. This makes it much more relaxing for those who struggle to concentrate or worry about 'doing it right', as many people working with stress or anxiety do.

These factors make Yoga Nidra a really accessible form of meditation. But 'more accessible' doesn't mean 'less powerful'. The states of meditation that we can reach through Yoga Nidra practice are equal to, if not even deeper than, standard sitting meditation practice.

~ *Sleep Notes* ~

For any pursed-lipped meditators out there calling heresy on what I said above, may I cheekily remind you that the Buddha himself taught lying-down meditation as one of the four main forms of mindfulness, equal in efficacy to the other three: sitting, walking and standing.

So, with the theory out of the way, let's learn how to practise Yoga Nidra and a variety of other hypnagogic mindfulness techniques.

CHAPTER 6

Rest and Relaxation
Practices

'Stress, no matter its source, is temporary
and does not reflect your true identity.'
JULIE T. LUSK, *YOGA NIDRA FOR COMPLETE*
RELAXATION AND STRESS RELIEF

A ll of the practices in this chapter create a shift towards
parasympathetic emphasis, which leads to reduced
stress and anxiety, deep relaxation and better sleep quality.
The Yoga Nidra and hypnagogic mindfulness practices in
particular are some of the easiest and most effective ways to
strengthen the relaxation response, calm the mind and create
a state of measurable neurological rest.

Exercise: Yoga Nidra

Yoga Nidra can be practised either during the day, in order to create
a habit of deep relaxation that will make it easier to fall asleep at
night, or at bedtime, as a precursor to sleep.

It can also be practised after waking up in the middle of the night as a way to make beneficial use of the time for relaxation or to relax ourselves back towards sleep.

For most people, the easiest way to practise Yoga Nidra is simply to follow a guided audio track while allowing yourself to drift through the hypnagogic. Many of these tracks are about 20–30 minutes long and will guide you through a relaxing body scan and encourage you to slow your breathing and often to imagine soothing imagery too.

There are loads of these audio tracks online and some can be a bit hit or miss, so for your convenience I've compiled a few of my favourites at www.charliemorley.com/wakeuptosleep.

The ones I personally recommend are from the iRest Institute, which specializes in trauma-sensitive Yoga Nidra, and Yoga Nidra Network, run by Uma Dinsmore-Tuli and her husband, Nirlipta, but find what works for you.

~ Select your Yoga Nidra audio track. I advise checking the volume level through your speaker or headphones before you begin the practice.

~ Prepare your space. This practice can be done sitting upright in a relaxed position, but ideally you would be lying down comfortably, usually on your back, either on the floor, on a sofa or in your bed. Most people like to have a pillow under their head and some people have a pillow under their knees too, to help relieve lower back pain. You want to feel totally comfortable, so use as many pillows, blankets and supports as you need. Unless you're doing this practice as a precursor to sleep, you don't want to be so comfortable that you black out, though, so be mindful of that.

~ Create some peace. Make sure your phone won't disturb you, but feel free to set an alarm to wake you at the end if you are worried about falling asleep during the practice. Do whatever needs to be done to allow you to relax more easily and, if necessary, tell anyone you share your space with what you're doing, so that they can act accordingly.

~ Play the audio track through your headphones or speaker and follow the instructions. If you fall asleep before the end, that's totally fine (and you will have got the benefits of a nap), but aim to stay deeply relaxed and aware within the hypnagogic state for the length of the track if possible.

~ Once the track has finished, don't rush back to waking life, but give yourself time to return gently, while still marinating in deep relaxation.

Daily Dosage

Either 20–30 minutes a day or twice a day, if possible, for those working with trauma or PTSD.

If that's not doable, then at least one 20-minute session three times per week, if you can.

You cannot overdose on this practice. On a Yoga Nidra retreat you might do six or seven 30-minute sessions per day and still sleep like a baby each night.

Exercise: Hypnagogic Mindfulness

This practice is very similar to Yoga Nidra, but it's self-guided rather than audio-track guided. It's a form of mindfulness meditation practised in the hypnagogic state that follows the 'Settling,

Grounding, Resting' protocol taught by a brilliant organization called the Mindfulness Association UK.

Owing to the mindful concentration required to guide yourself into the hypnogogic without blacking out, it may not be quite as relaxing as an audio-guided Yoga Nidra session. However, because it follows a mindfulness meditation format, it has the same amazing neurological benefits as standard mindfulness meditation, such as an increase in the grey-matter density of the hippocampus (an area responsible for learning and memory) and decreased density in the amygdala (an area responsible for anxiety and stress responses).[1]

Just like Yoga Nidra, hypnogogic mindfulness can be practised either during the day or at night, and it's great for when you don't have access to an audio track or if you'd simply prefer to guide yourself.

~ Prepare your space. This practice can be done sitting upright in a relaxed position, but ideally you would be lying down comfortably, usually on your back, either on the floor, on a sofa or in your bed. Most people like to have a pillow under their head and some people have a pillow under their knees too, to help relieve lower back pain. You want to feel totally comfortable, so use as many pillows, blankets and supports as you need. Unless you are doing this practice as a precursor to sleep, you don't want to be so comfortable that you black out instantly, though, so be mindful of that.

~ Do whatever needs to be done to allow you to relax more easily and then read through the instructions below to roughly memorize the different stages of the practice.

~ If you aren't using the practice as a precursor to sleep, set a gentle-sounding alarm for 20–30 minutes later.

~ Close your eyes and relax.

~ Become aware of your breathing and then proceed to settle your mind by breathing in for a count of three or four and breathing out for a count of three or four.

~ Continue breathing this way for a few minutes. When you have thoughts, just let them go freely, without attempting to reject or engage them. Simply leave them be and bring your focus back to the breathing and counting.

~ After a few minutes, begin to focus a little more on the out-breath. Notice that as you release the out-breath, your body relaxes a little more.

~ And then feel free to drop the breath counting.

~ Now, breathing naturally, begin to ground yourself by bringing your awareness into your body. Simply become aware of all the bodily sensations you are experiencing. That's all. Feel the contact between your body and the ground beneath it. Feel the weight of your body and relax into the unconditional support of the ground. Then begin scanning your awareness from the tips of your toes to the crown of your head (a full-body scan), relaxing deeply as you go. Take at least 10 minutes for this if you can, or continue until your entire body has relaxed into awareness.

~ Now, simply rest. Don't do anything. Drop any idea of trying to do anything. Just rest. Simply rest in the moment. Be aware of whatever comes to you. If you feel yourself starting to slip into sleep, bring your attention back to the flow of your breath, the sounds in the room and your contact with the surface beneath you. If you feel that you are about to black out, you might like to lightly contract your fingers or toes as a way of bringing yourself back to bodily awareness.

~ Allow yourself to rest in this mindful awareness of the hypnagogic state for the rest of your session. When the mind drifts off, use awareness of your breath or the hypnagogic imagery to bring yourself back to the present moment.

~ Either end your practice when your alarm goes off or allow yourself to slip into sleep if you are using this practice as a precursor to sleep.

I have my own 25-minute guided audio-track version of this practice called 'The Dao of Dozing', taken from an album of guided audio meditations called *Lucid Dreaming, Conscious Sleeping* that can be downloaded from iTunes or Audible.com.

Daily Dosage

This can be done instead of or alongside your Yoga Nidra practice, but aim for at least 20–30 minutes a day of either one, or twice a day if you are working with trauma or PTSD.

If that's not doable, then at least one 20-minute session three times per week if you can.

► Field-Tested Feedback

Yoga Nidra and hypnagogic mindfulness are among the most popular exercises for workshop participants. I'm often asked to explain the science behind them over and over again, because people struggle to accept that something so relaxing and so enjoyable can actually be good for them! This is truly a testament to the lost regard of the sacred nature of rest.

Feedback from a workshop I ran that included women from the Army Widows' Association beautifully stated: 'I'd never come across this before as a practice in its own right. I just thought it was the 'best bit' at the end of yoga classes. To meditate lying down with the body utterly at ease is a joy and makes so much sense. And the quality of communion with something sacred-seeming is more precious than gold.'

And: 'The Yoga Nidra practice instantly changed me for the better. I feel much more grounded as a result and am hopeful that it will penetrate the deeper levels of nervousness and anxiety in my nervous system over time. I have not missed a day of practice since learning this technique.'

One woman said: 'It's very restorative and practical. It recharges the batteries, and when I do it in my lunch break, I have a much better afternoon at work.'

One of the benefits of hypnagogic mindfulness and Yoga Nidra that people come back to again and again is that it offers them something to do if they wake up in the middle of the night and can't get back to sleep. It is a great way to either relax back into sleep or at least to use the wakeful period for deep, neurologically beneficial rest rather than the energy-consuming, ANS-activating process of 'trying to sleep'. Essentially, five hours' sleep plus half an hour of deep rest is way better than five hours' sleep plus two hours of stressfully trying to force ourselves back to sleep!

•••

The exercises below should be used alongside (not instead of) your daily practice of either Yoga Nidra or hypnagogic mindfulness if possible.

Exercise: Hypnagogic Affirmations for Quality Sleep

This one is a bit of a 'love it/hate it' technique, but for some people it can be really helpful for reprogramming their limiting beliefs around sleep.

An affirmation is simply a positive declaration of intent. Reading affirmations or saying them out loud can have a powerful effect on our mental state, and if we say them in the alpha and theta-rich hypnotic trance-state of the hypnagogic, this effect is supercharged.

Author Jennifer Williamson has written a book about this called *Sleep Affirmations*, in which she explains how affirmations are great tools for interrupting negative thought patterns and for strengthening the beliefs that serve us.

A couple of my favourite affirmations from her are:

I am totally worthy of the sleep I seek.

May my sleep be peaceful. May my dreams be filled with love.

Here are a few others that you might like to try too:

I release today and relax deeply into sleep.

May my sleep be peaceful and my mind at ease.

All is well. I am safe and relaxed.

Nothing to do, nowhere to go, resting.

By repeating one of these affirmations as you drift off to sleep, you are letting your body know that you're safe, and that it's okay to receive the rest that is your birthright.

~   Choose an affirmation or create your own.

~   Repeat it a handful of times while fully awake to learn it off by heart and to allow the underlying energy of the words to take root.

~   Lie down in bed and close your eyes. Once you begin drifting into the hypnagogic state, repeat your affirmation mindfully and with feeling.

~   After a few minutes of repeating the affirmation, allow yourself to fall asleep, saturated with the beneficial energy of the words.

Daily Dosage

As and when you like.

This technique is particularly good if you are struggling to pass through the hypnogogic either first thing at night or after a night-time awakening.

Feel free to combine it with hypnagogic mindfulness too.

Exercise: Progressive Muscular Relaxation

Dr Edmund Jacobson invented this technique way back in the 1920s as a way of helping his patients deal with anxiety. He was a man ahead of his time, who knew that relaxing the muscles of the body could relax the mind as well.

The technique simply involves working through various muscle groups, first tensing and then releasing them. It usually starts with the feet and then works up through the body slowly and smoothly.

By tensing and releasing specific areas of our body, we not only become more aware of our body (which is great for counteracting dissociation), but also more aware of the tension we have been holding.

Often people have been stressed out for so long that they don't actually know that they're tense. But if you ask them to intentionally *create tension* and then release it, a new-found awareness of what relaxation feels like can be experienced and absorbed.

This technique can be done at any time of day or night, but if we practise it while we're drifting through the hypnagogic, it may lead to an even deeper level of relaxation.

~ Prepare your space. This practice can be done sitting upright in a relaxed position, but ideally you would be lying down comfortably, usually on your back, either on the floor, on a sofa or in your bed. Close your eyes and adjust your body so that you are as comfortable as possible.

~ While inhaling through your nose, tense each muscle group in turn (*see below*), quite strongly but without discomfort, for about five counts, then release the tension in that muscle group as you exhale for about eight to ten counts. Feel the tension draining away from those muscles. Let them feel heavy and relaxed. Give yourself ten counts or so to relax, and then move on to the next muscle group. Gradually work your way up your body, tensing and releasing each of the following muscle groups in turn:

• feet and ankles

• lower legs

- upper legs

- hips, lower back and glutes

- abdomen and chest

- hands and arms

- shoulders and neck

- face (scrunch it up)

- entire body

While releasing the tension, try to focus on how you feel when the muscle group is released and relaxed. Feel free to imagine that stressful feelings are flowing out of your body as you relax each muscle group too.

~ Repeat the very last step (full-body tensing) three times and allow your entire body to feel heavy and relaxed. Let go of any residual tension and imagine it flowing out of your body as you sink into deep relaxation.

~ Enjoy the feelings of relaxation for a few more moments and then allow yourself to either drift off to sleep or open your eyes and stretch into full wakefulness.

Daily Dosage

As and when you like.

Particularly good for restless leg syndrome or discharging stress from a day either without much movement or with loads of it (perhaps after a long run or a gym workout).

Exercise: Napping

Hypnagogic mindfulness and Yoga Nidra are great ways to recharge our batteries and rest deeply without actually sleeping. Sometimes, though, we might actually want to catch up on some proper sleep or simply add to our daily quota, and as long as it's done at least six hours before we intend to go to bed, napping can be a great way to do that.

Let's not forget: the seven to nine hours *per night* should actually be read as *per 24-hour period*, as it is in many siesta-loving countries, and so napping absolutely counts towards your daily sleep quota and is often a much more realistic way of boosting your sleep time than trying to stay in bed for eight hours straight at night.

Interestingly, when we nap outside of our nightly monophasic sleep, the sleep stage sequence is different and deep sleep comes after light sleep and REM. This also makes napping great for the lucid dreaming practices we will learn later.

THE SCIENCE OF NAPS

Psychology professor Kimberly A. Cote says, 'If you're talking about the healthy adult population, I think just about anyone could benefit from a nap.'[2]

A six-year Harvard Medical School study has shown that those who nap regularly are 37 per cent less likely to die of heart disease than non-nappers, with male nappers reducing their chance of heart disease even more, by up to 64 per cent.[3] There is no daily medicine that can reduce a man's chances of dying from heart disease by that much, so naps do offer really quite incredible results.

A sleepless night can increase irritability (due to over-reactivity in the brain's threat detector, the amygdala) by up to 60 per cent, but thankfully a 60-minute nap can greatly reduce that reactivity[4] and even naps as short as 20–30 minutes can decrease fatigue and improve mood and alertness. In fact, a study at NASA found that a 40-minute nap improved astronauts' alertness by up to 100 per cent, while improving their overall performance by 34 per cent.[5]

The most fascinating fact that I know about naps was discovered by Dr Sara Mednick, a psychologist at the University of California, who found that after a 60–90-minute afternoon nap, people performed just as well on a memory test as they did after a full night of sleep. She said, 'It's amazing. In a 90-minute nap, you can get the same learning benefits as in an eight-hour sleep period.'[6]

I don't want to labour the point here, but napping is incredibly good for you and makes you measurably better at whatever you do after it, so I highly recommend finding a way to bring it into your daily or weekly routine.

~ Sleep Notes ~

Why napping isn't integrated into our education, work and societal structures is beyond me. Students could be getting better grades, stock market traders could be making better trades and politicians could be making better-informed (and fewer amygdala-affected) decisions if they were all given the space to have an hour's nap each day.

Top Tips for Napping

- Although most people feel the urge to nap around mid-afternoon, feel free to nap whenever you like, as long as it's at least six hours before you intend to go to bed. This is in order to give your body enough time to build up its 'sleep pressure', the biological basis of tiredness, before bedtime.

- If you do feel the need for a recharge later in the evening, opt for a Yoga Nidra session instead, as this won't adversely affect your sleep pressure.

- Most people find that a nap of between 20 and 90 minutes is best.

- Try not to nap for much more than 90 minutes, though. Anything over that may lead you into delta-wave sleep (remember, the sleep stage sequence is different in naps), which might make you feel a bit groggy when you wake up and negatively affect your sleep that night.

If you can't nap, then at least rest. In his book *Sleep*, elite sports sleep coach Nick Littlehales recommends his athletes take a 90-minute controlled recovery period (CRP) every day. This could be as much as a full-on 90-minute sleep, as little a 60–90-minute eyes-open rest in a darkened room, or anything in between. The point is to allow the body to do nothing other than rest, recover and relax for 90 minutes at least once a day.

CHAPTER 7

Trauma and PTSD

*'Trauma is hell on Earth. Trauma
resolved is a gift from the gods.'*

PETER A. LEVINE, DEVELOPER OF SOMATIC EXPERIENCING®

We could have explored this topic much earlier, but in order to be as 'trauma sensitive' as possible, I wanted to wait until we had some of the tools to help integrate trauma before delving into it.

Trauma and post-traumatic stress disorder (PTSD) are usually associated with life-threatening events such as war, rape, physical and sexual abuse, natural disasters, violence or accidents, but it's important to know that, as mentioned earlier, we can also be traumatized by events that might seem much more mundane. Traumatization is created by any experience that overwhelms our ability to cope, and that can include inadequate parenting, heartbreak, bullying at school or work and social media abuse. People sometimes think that their trauma 'isn'tenough' to take seriously, but trauma is trauma, whether from a military warzone or the warzone of a family home.

Post-Traumatic Stress

Post-traumatic stress is a totally normal response to a traumatic experience. As we go through a traumatic incident, almost all of us will experience a high level of distress and fear. This has an 'aftershock' effect on our nervous system, which might result in nightmares, anxiety, depression or feeling scared to visit the place where the incident occurred or to do the activity that led to the trauma.

This is a hardwired part of our physiology and totally natural. James Scurry, a mindfulness-based psychotherapist specializing in trauma, agrees: 'Post-traumatic stress happens to everybody. We so often pathologize things like nightmares, depression and anxiety, but the process of experiencing trauma after something traumatizing is part of what makes us human.'[1]

Much of the time, just as with physical wounds, our body's innate healing capacity naturally integrates our psychological trauma and so usually post-traumatic stress symptoms fade away within a few days or weeks of the traumatic incident without the need for either drugs or therapy. Just as a naturally healed physical wound sometimes leaves a scar, so too do our psychological wounds. However, if we learn how to release and integrate even small traumas, we can learn to heal without being scarred.

Sometimes, though, a certain trauma hits much harder: we feel it much more deeply, it lasts much longer and affects us more acutely. We might have flashbacks, when we relive or re-experience aspects of the trauma, or high levels of anxiety and hypervigilance, recurring nightmares, significant behavioural changes, crippling depression and numbing or dissociation that not only overwhelm our ability to cope but, crucially, don't seem to fade with time. This is when our experience might start to meet the criteria of PTSD.

Post-Traumatic Stress Disorder

Although it depends on the type of trauma experienced, in general only about 16 per cent of traumatized people will develop symptoms that meet the criteria of clinical PTSD,[2] whereas many others might have hugely distressing and potentially life-disabling symptoms and yet be classed as having 'sub-clinical' PTSD. For some, the diagnosis of PTSD can be a blessing, as it provides a helpful label to explain what they have been going through, while for others it becomes a heavy burden of perceived shame or brokenness.

This book isn't designed for any form of self-diagnosis, so be sure to seek help and guidance from medical professionals if more information about PTSD would be helpful to you.

All of the techniques in the book have been successfully taught both to groups with high levels of PTSD and groups with none, so we know that they can be helpful for everyone, regardless.

Whatever label we give it, it's important to know that the effects of trauma can lie dormant within us for years, even decades after the traumatic event. Some describe this as being like a silently ticking time-bomb that finally detonates when a triggering event – the 10-year anniversary of the trauma, a song on the radio that was playing at the time, or simply a stressful life change such as retirement or childbirth – sets it off.

The good news is that we *can* defuse the time-bomb. Working with a body-based approach to trauma can allow for the healing and integration of hidden or latent past trauma before the bomb goes off. We're not destined to explode; we're destined to heal.

Trauma isn't our fault, but responding to it is our responsibility, and our 'ability to respond' begins the moment we understand three crucial points about trauma:

1. Being traumatized or having PTSD isn't a sign of weakness; in fact, it's often those who push themselves the hardest and feel the deepest who suffer the worst.

2. Trauma is neurological, not just psychological, meaning that we can't 'just get over it', however much we cognitively try to do so.

3. Understanding how trauma dysregulates our brain can be used to help destigmatize its effects and bring ourselves back into balance.

When I asked my friend Cliff Grady, a Vietnam veteran who now works as a therapist in San Francisco, how we could best help people with trauma, he told me: 'Believe them. Believe their pain. You can't always see wounds. Some wounds, like PTSD, are invisible, but they are terrible. So, even if the traumatized person can't verbalize it, at least be willing to see it.'[3]

Three Women in an Office: How Trauma Affects the Brain

Dr Heather Sequeira is a brilliant consultant psychologist who specializes in working with trauma.[4] At one of her PTSD Masterclasses that I attended in London, she explained how the brain is changed by trauma by using the scenario of three women in an office.

Each woman works in a separate department and represents a different part of the brain.

First of all, we have Mrs Cortex, who represents the prefrontal cortex part of the brain. Mrs Cortex is the boss and CEO. She is very clever. She is a decision-maker, a stickler for time-keeping, an expert in abstract thought and a brilliant problem-solver. She makes predictions about future events and is a lover of words and linguistics.

Next we have Ms Hippocampus, who represents the part of the brain called the hippocampus. Ms Hippocampus is the personal assistant of Mrs Cortex. She is a great organizer, does all the filing, works the computer systems and is especially skilled at data storage. She works very closely with Mrs Cortex, showing her new information and then filing it away where her boss can make sense of it.

And finally we have Mary Amygdala, who represents the part of the brain called the amygdala. Mary looks after the front desk; she is a receptionist cum security guard. She screens visitors, checks the CCTV and, crucially, controls the office alarm system. She does her job well, but she isn't that bright and tends to think in black and white terms.

A Man in a Hat

One day a man wearing a hat and waving a loaded gun walks into the office. Mary Amygdala, thank goodness, sees the threat, hits the alarm button and automatically locks the doors to the departments of the boss, Mrs Cortex, and her assistant, Ms Hippocampus. Mary is doing her job as best she can and following protocol. Once she locks the doors, the decision-making capacity of Mrs Cortex is blocked and the internal data-filing capacity of Ms Hippocampus is offline, but at least Mary Amygdala can concentrate on protecting the office and letting the security forces (the 'fight or flight' systems) know how to proceed.

Once the threat has been dealt with, she reopens the phone lines, unlocks the doors to the other departments, and the office can start returning to normal.

Crucially, though, Mrs Cortex and Ms Hippocampus were locked down during the whole incident, so they didn't have any influence over what happened and they didn't actually get much information about the man with the gun either. The whole traumatic experience is stored in the reception area of Mary Amygdala.

Another Man in a Hat

A month later, another man in a hat walks into the office. He does *not* have a gun and poses no threat, but because Mary Amygdala thinks in black and white terms and doesn't have the same level of rational intelligence as her boss, Mrs Cortex, she assumes that *anyone* wearing a hat is a threat.

What should she do? She could phone through to her boss to ask, but it might take too long and she can't risk it. She's still affected by what happened last month and she's been on edge ever since. So she activates the alarm system, locks down the other departments and cuts the phone lines too, just as she did last time.

The Three Women in an Office metaphor describes a totally normal response from a brain affected by trauma, but let's break it down step by step.

Once we have experienced a traumatic event at the hands of 'a man in a hat waving a loaded gun', it's totally normal that the next time we see 'a man in a hat', our amygdala alarm system will be activated automatically. It's not our fault, it's just the way our brain has been affected by trauma: *we respond to a present situation based on the memory of a past threat.*

As we reflect on a traumatic experience we've been through, we might ask ourselves, 'Why did I make such crazy decisions?' or 'Why didn't I fight back?' or 'Why can't I remember what they looked like?'

The reason we often make irrational decisions during a traumatic event, or make no decision at all and simply freeze, is because the part of our brain that makes rational decisions is offline. Mary Amygdala has shut down access to the higher reasoning and decision-making capacities of Mrs Cortex.

She has also cut the lines of communication to Ms Hippocampus, so our memory and data-storage capacity are offline too. That's why we often struggle to remember the exact details or timeline of a traumatic experience. It's not our fault, it's simply a product of our brain activity.

So, if you've been carrying guilt about the way you reacted during a traumatic experience or the disordered memories you have about it, let me tell you this personally: *it is not your fault.*

~ *Sleep Notes* ~

No wonder you couldn't remember what the person looked like: your hippocampus was offline. No wonder you didn't make rational decisions: your prefrontal cortex was offline. No wonder you didn't fight back: your amygdala had put you into freeze response. Once we understand that, we can stop blaming ourselves for how we reacted and start to move towards healing.

THE SCIENCE OF FLASHBACKS

Sometimes a traumatic event can have such a strong impact on our brain that afterwards we re-experience aspects of it. When this happens during the day, we call it a 'flashback', and if it happens while we are asleep, it manifests as a nightmare or night terror. (More on these in Chapters 11 and 12.)

Flashbacks are usually caused by a trigger – something that subconsciously reminds us of the trauma. They aren't just intrusive memories, they are a visceral re-experiencing of the trauma. Using our 'Three women in an office' metaphor, a flashback would make Mary Amygdala go through exactly the same procedure of locking down the office and setting off the alarm system *as if there actually was* a man in a hat waving a gun in her face.

Neuroimaging studies[5] confirm that during a flashback both the prefrontal cortex and the hippocampus really do go offline, which is why, just like the trauma that they are replaying, flashbacks are often so difficult to recall coherently or be rationally talked out of.

Dr Bessel van der Kolk, author of the seminal *The Body Keeps the Score*, was among the first to state that trauma could only be fully integrated once the brain structures that were knocked out during the traumatic experience were brought fully back online and the traumatic imprint on the brain was integrated. This was at a time when the mainstream scientific establishment was still trying to 'talk away' trauma and many were unwilling to open up to his revolutionary and now well-accepted work. If any book has had the greatest impact on my writing this one, it is *The Body Keeps the Score* – a highly recommended read.

Wellbeing in the Workplace

After a traumatic event, our brain may well be physiologically changed. A 2020 meta-analysis of over 50 papers on PTSD found that trauma led to a reduction in prefrontal cortex thickness and hippocampal volume, as well as to an increase in amygdala activity.[6]

So how do we counteract the neurological effects of trauma and get those three women in the office working well again?

There are three main ways:

1. recalibrate the dysregulated amygdala (through breath and bodywork practices)

2. strengthen the capacity of the prefrontal cortex (through mindfulness practices)

3. calm the hippocampus by reducing the levels of cortisol in the body[7] (through rest and relaxation practices)

Recalibrating the Amygdala

Mary Amygdala is a kinaesthetic learner, so she responds best to movement and breath practices. The body-scanning aspect of Yoga Nidra and the breathwork with movement practices of Breath-Body-Mind, which we will look at in Chapter 10, are exactly what she needs in order to recalibrate.

Studies from Harvard researchers[8] showed that just 30 minutes of mindfulness practice a day decreased the grey-matter density (and the reactivity of) the amygdala within just four weeks, so all forms of mindfulness are great for Mary too.

Once Mary Amygdala is chilled out and healthy, she will gladly open up the phone lines to Mrs Cortex and the rational thinking required for remedies like cognitive behavioural therapy (CBT) and talk therapy, but until then they might not be that effective.

Strengthening the Prefrontal Cortex

The easiest way to do this is to practise any form of mindfulness or awareness training.

Mindfulness leads directly to increased thickness in the prefrontal cortex,[9] which in turn strengthens its capacity for insight, rational thinking and executive function. Basically, the way to refurbish the office of Mrs Cortex is to regularly practise mindfulness. Whether you choose standard sitting mindfulness (great for some, but not so ideal for those working with trauma), hypnagogic mindfulness or the Coherent Breathing and the Breath-Body-Mind practices of the next few chapters, all have the same beneficial effect.

We want to strengthen the capacity of the prefrontal cortex not only to increase our capacity for self-regulation, but also to dial down the reactivity of the amygdala. This is because it's a bi-directional relationship, so once Mrs Cortex is back online she can start advising Mary on her meet-and-greet strategy.

Calming the Hippocampus

The effects of trauma on the ANS keep the levels of stress hormones abnormally high. This has a harmful effect on the hippocampus and can even cause Ms Hippocampus to 'call in sick', meaning that flashbacks and nightmares continue, because the memories of the trauma can't be processed.

Once cortisol and adrenaline levels get back to normal, Ms Hippocampus can start doing her job again: processing the trauma and filing away the disturbing memories.

How best to do that? Relaxation and mindfulness. The 'rest and relax' practices of the previous chapter are a great way to start. Deep relaxation and mindfulness practices in general can lead to a 50 per cent reduction in cortisol levels[10] and increases in grey-matter density of the hippocampus.[11]

The body-based, stress-reducing mindfulness practices in this book have been specifically curated to recalibrate the amygdala, strengthen the prefrontal cortex and calm the hippocampus, giving you the best chance of getting those three women in an office back into perfect balance.

And of course, once your brain is in balance, your sleep will be too.

Post-Traumatic Growth

I want to end this chapter by exploring the fascinating field of post-traumatic growth (PTG). This refers to the phenomenon of positive change that is made following an experience of trauma and adversity.

Just as there is a scale for measuring PTSD, so there is one for measuring PTG, which includes changes in the appreciation of life, relationships with others, personal strength and even spiritual outlook.

There is a Tibetan saying that seems to refer to something similar: 'Just as a bonfire in a strong wind is not blown out, but blazes even brighter, so our mind can be strengthened by the difficult situations we encounter.'

Amazingly, more than half of all trauma survivors actually report experiencing positive change once the initial aftershocks of the trauma have passed.[12] A 2009 *British Journal of Health Psychology* article reviewing the past 20 years of studies into PTG reported: 'The studies consistently found that their respondents had a new appreciation of life, calling it a "gift", and that they were even thankful that they had been touched by such life-altering illnesses or events.'[13]

Psychologists agree that 'Following the acute period of depression, anxiety or nightmares caused by the trauma, we can arrive at an even higher level of psychological and emotional functioning than before the adversity.'[14] Researchers commented how people said that 'despite the physical pain they suffered and the daily struggles they faced, their lives were unquestionably better today than before their traumatic experiences. Trauma sent them on a path they never would have found otherwise.'[15]

Of course this wasn't true of all traumatized people: although about 50 per cent reported PTG, that still leaves 50 per cent without it, struggling to integrate their trauma.

My inclusion of PTG in this chapter is not to minimize the devastating impact of traumatization, but simply to let you know that PTG is a possibility. Also, just like PTSD, it can take years for PTG to manifest, so we never know whether psychological growth is just round the corner.

There is a Buddhist metaphor that encapsulates the essence of PTG perfectly: 'No mud, no lotus.'

No Mud, No Lotus

In the Buddhist tradition, the lotus flower is a symbol of our innate potential for enlightenment. The reason for this stems from how the lotus grows. Lotus seeds grow most readily in the deep sludge at the bottom of ponds. When they sprout, they are naturally attracted to the sunlight that shines down through the murky water and instinctively reach up to it, eventually blossoming above the surface of the water, pristine, perfect and beautiful, untainted by the mud from whence they came.

Buddhist thought tells us that the lotus flower is like our true human potential and the muddy pond is like our confused, stressed and traumatized mind. All the painful, shameful, and traumatic aspects of both our mind and our life form the fertile mud in which the lotus can grow. Without the mud, there can be no lotus. The mud is a prerequisite for psycho-spiritual growth.

The first time I came across this concept, I was amazed to learn that my traumatized, shameful, seemingly 'muddy' mind-states might actually be instigating or igniting psychological growth. And now the concept allows me to see clearly that my mum's Alzheimer's has bonded me more closely to my brother, taught me patience and allowed me to love my mum unconditionally, and that the end of my marriage has forced me to face, embrace and transform the crippling fear of loneliness that had limited me for so long.

Perhaps there has been a time in your life when the mud of suffering has led to the lotus of psychological growth?

When I've introduced the 'no mud, no lotus' metaphor at workshops, people have shared how losing their job led them to the career they'd always dreamed of, how mental breakdown led them to the spiritual path and how illness was the wake-up call that led to living a fuller life.

The 'no mud, no lotus' idea isn't about spiritual bypassing and 'seeing the bright side', but simply about acknowledging that sometimes our trauma, however painful, can fertilize the seeds of our personal growth. This can take years to come to fruition, but it very often does.

Part II Checklist ✓

✓ Give yourself permission to rest and relax. Nobody deserves it more than you.

✓ Practise hypnagogic mindfulness or Yoga Nidra for 20–30 minutes every day, or at least three times a week if possible. Anything is better than nothing though, so even just one session a week will offer noticeable benefits.

✓ Don't forget to keep up your Nocturnal Journal.

✓ Learn the basics of the 'Three women in an office' metaphor as a way to help destigmatize trauma and remind yourself that your behaviour both during and after a traumatic event is not your fault, but the product of a brain in survival mode.

✓ Notice any changes to your sleep cycle that might result from the hypnagogic mindfulness or Yoga Nidra practices.

✓ Close your mouth. You'll find out why in the next chapter.

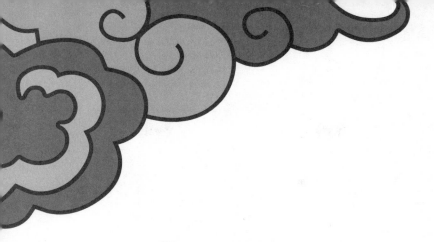

PART III

AND BREATHE...

*'If I had to limit my advice on healthier living to just
one tip, it would be to learn to breathe correctly.'*

DR ANDREW WEIL, PIONEER IN THE FIELD OF INTEGRATIVE MEDICINE

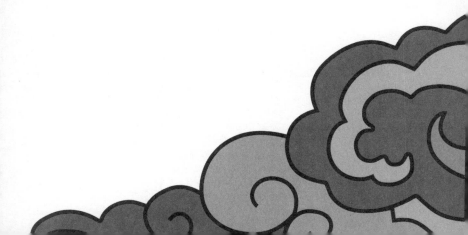

Now that we've learned how to relax and explored how trauma works, it's time to turn our attention to our breathing. It's the thing that we are constantly doing, both awake and asleep, yet the thing that most of us aren't doing quite right.

In this part of the book we'll explore how changing the way we breathe can have a powerful impact on regulating our nervous system, integrating trauma and allowing us to sleep soundly.

Just as we need to relearn how to sleep, so we need to relearn how to breathe.

CHAPTER 8

Breathe Right

*'Deep breathing changes the chemistry of
the body. So, breathe, motherfuckers!'*
WIM HOFF

As shamans, mystics and yogis have known for thousands of years, we can radically transform our psycho-physical state through the rhythm of our breath.

Breathing practices have been used within various lineages of yoga, martial arts and meditation as a way of raising energy levels, balancing the neurological system and lengthening life. Western science is now finally catching up to the fact that controlled breathing practices can at least 'enhance immunity, improve cardiovascular fitness, modulate chronic disease and increase longevity',[1] and at most lead to almost superhuman feats. From Wim Hoff stimulating his immune system to repel E. coli to Dr Stan Grof using hyperventilation to create hallucinatory head-trips to Harvard Medical School proving that Tibetan monks can dry wet sheets by voluntarily increasing their body heat,[2] we now have hard science to prove that breathing practices can produce seemingly miraculous results.

The reason why changing the way we breathe can have such a profound impact on our physiology is because the brain fast tracks messages from the lungs above all others.

The Brain Has the Lungs on Speed Dial

Over thousands of years of evolution, fast and powerful pathways between the respiratory system and the brain have been established. If breathing stops, death occurs within minutes, and so the brain prioritizes messages from the lungs above all others.

In fact, as breathwork expert Dr Pat Gerbarg says, the brain never stops listening to the lungs. Medical research has shown that 'messages from the respiratory system have rapid, powerful effects on major brain centres involved in thought, emotion and behaviour'.[3]

You may have noticed that when you see something shocking, you might inhale sharply, or when you sink into your favourite spot on the sofa, you might exhale deeply, right? So you already know that specific emotional responses induce specific breathing patterns. But what you may not have noticed is that it works the other way round too: we can induce specific emotions by breathing in a certain way.[4]

Our breathing pattern can have an enormous effect on our psycho-physical state. This means that changing the way we breathe can literally change the way we feel, almost instant-aneously. Want to be relaxed? Breathe like you already are.

Optimize Your Breathing

In the introduction to his brilliantly researched book *Breath: The New Science of a Lost Art*, James Nestor reckons that 90 per cent of us are breathing incorrectly[5] and that sub-optimal breathing lies at the core of a whole host of medical conditions.

Breathwork pioneer Stephen Elliott agrees, saying, 'Myriad health problems and the huge rates of heart disease, Alzheimer's, diabetes and sleeplessness may well be fundamentally rooted in the fact that we have never been taught how to breathe correctly.'[6]

But how can we breathe *in*correctly? Surely breathing is automatic?

Breathing, just like sleep, *is* an automatic function, but one that, just like sleep, has become autonomously sub-optimized due to both environmental and psycho-physical stressors.

Just as learning how to sleep intentionally can transform one-third of our life, learning how to breathe intentionally can transform the other two-thirds. Over the next couple of chapters we're going to learn some breathing techniques that have been proven to help integrate stress and trauma and reduce insomnia. But before that, let's explore three simple adjustments through which we can optimize our everyday breathing habits.

Shut Your Mouth

Breathing through your mouth is bad for you. Around 50 per cent of Americans are habitual mouth-breathers[7] and there is growing evidence to suggest that the epidemic of sleep problems facing Americans may be directly linked to this fact. This is because how we breathe while awake dictates how we breathe while we sleep.

Breathing through your nose, however, is really good for you. The nose has a three-layer filtration system made up of nasal hairs, which help stop dirt and debris entering the respiratory system, a mucus membrane, which catches dust and bacteria before they enter the lungs, and finally microscopic hairs called cilia, which help move the mucus along the respiratory tract and further filter out the bad stuff.

Mouth breathing has no such three-layer filtration system, meaning that germs, allergens and other pollutants can get inside our lungs, where they can damage delicate tissues.

Our nose not only filters the air we breathe in, but also heats or cools and humidifies it in the nasal cavity (which is actually greater in volume than our mouth cavity, amazingly), making it easier for our lungs to absorb.

~ Sleep Notes ~

How to tell if you're a night-time mouth-breather? If you wake up with a dry mouth or feel thirsty in the middle of the night, then you are probably breathing through your mouth. And if you snore regularly, you almost certainly are.

Fascinatingly, nasal breathing actually increases our oxygen intake too. When I first heard this, I found it very hard to believe. I knew from my kickboxing days that during a fight I would instinctively want to breathe through my mouth to try to give my body the increased level of oxygen that it was craving, but it turns out that although mouth breathing may seem to bring in more air, it doesn't actually bring in more oxygen.

Nasal breathing not only increases the vacuum in the lungs, which allows us to draw in 20 per cent more oxygen than breathing through the mouth, but it also increases nitric oxide release from the sinuses, meaning that 18 per cent more of that extra oxygen can be absorbed.[8]

Higher nitric oxide levels increase blood circulation and oxygen delivery to all cells in the body, and simply by breathing in through our nose, we can increase nitric oxide levels by up to 600 per cent.[9] Nitric oxide is antifungal, antiviral, antiparasitic and antibacterial, so nasal breathing does way more than just filter the air.

Mouth breathing also makes us less smart. A 2019 Japanese study[10] found that rats that had their nostrils plugged and were forced to breathe through their mouths developed fewer brain cells and were so cognitively impaired that they took double the time to find cheese in a maze.

And finally, mouth breathing is also really bad for our teeth. It contributes to gum disease and bad breath, and is believed by some dentists to be the leading cause of cavities, above even sugar consumption and a bad diet.[11]

~ *Sleep Notes* ~

People often wonder about exhaling through their mouth. This is fine, but exhaling through the nose is often even better, as doing so helps to expel the trapped particles and bacteria that the nasal cavity has caught on the inhale.

So, how can we be sure to inhale through our nose as much as possible? There are three main ways:

- Every time you notice that you're mouth breathing, or even simply that your mouth is open, close it so that you have to breathe through your nose.

- Do at least 20 minutes of conscious breathwork a day as a way of becoming more mindful about how you breathe and to create a new habit of nasal inhalation.

- Consider mouth-taping at night (yup, it's a thing), so that you are nasal breathing for a third of your life at least. Although this sounds like quite a radical intervention and it's definitely not for everyone, it has loads of science to back it up and can be a real game-changer for some people. If you are going to try mouth-taping, though, it's important to know that the aim is not to hermetically seal your mouth shut, but simply to encourage nasal breathing by making mouth breathing more difficult to do. How? By placing a small vertical strip of surgical tape over the midline of your lips and keeping it there while you sleep. Check www.charliemorley.com/wakeuptosleep for a demonstration of mouth-taping.

Expand Your Lungs

The second way to optimize your breathing is to intentionally expand your lungs so that breathing can happen more effectively.

A 30-year study from the State University of New York at Buffalo with more than 1,000 subjects found that larger lungs equalled longer lives[12] and that lung capacity was one of the greatest indicators of longevity.

In these post-pandemic times, our lung capacity is becoming increasing important, as it is directly linked to our ability to recover from respiratory infections such as covid-19. As the lead researcher of the Buffalo study said, 'The lung is a primary defence organism against environmental toxins,'[13] so healthy lungs can mean the difference between life and death.

What do we actually need to do to expand our lung capacity? Slow, deep breathing, and lots of it.

A 2020 medical study poetically titled 'Equanimity in the time of COVID' found: 'Slow, deep breathing can increase the volume of the lungs by a massive 600 per cent, while increasing the surface area of the lungs by up to 30 per cent.'[14]

Slow Down

As you read these words, you're probably breathing at around about 15 breaths per minute. This might seem normal, but it is actually so fast that it activates the sympathetic nervous system. This means that right now, simply because of the way you are breathing, your body is in low-level 'fight or flight' mode. No wonder so many of us feel anxious all the time: our body is on red alert even while we're reading a book.

This not only plays havoc with our ability to sleep well, as it activates the release of the cortisol, adrenaline and excitatory neurotransmitters that keep us awake, but, as we learned earlier, it also exacerbates, and contributes to, a whole host of illnesses, including heart disease, cancer and chronic inflammation.

So how can we counteract this constant activation of our 'fight or flight' system while also expanding our lung capacity? By simply breathing much, much more slowly than usual. In the next chapter we'll learn a breathing technique that will slow our breathing from around 15 breaths per minute to five. That may seem incredibly slow, but it's actually a very natural way to breathe. In fact, it's the way we were breathing until very recently. Forrest Knutson, author of *Hacking the Universe: The Process of Yogic Meditation*, has done brilliant research into the varying average breath rates of the 20th century. In one of his videos he references a State University of New York at Buffalo study that found the average breath rate of American adults in 1929 was just 4.9 breaths per minute.[15] That's a whopping 70 per cent slower than today.

Another study found the average breath rate in 1939 to be just 5.3 breaths per minute.[16] In 1950, with the growing popularization of mod-cons and processed food, and the more sedentary lifestyles of office work and TV watching, as well as the traumatic aftermath of WWII, the average breath rate jumped to 6.9 BPM.[17] But even as recently as 1980, it was still as low as 7.8 breaths per minute.[18]

In the year 2020 the average adult breath rate had jumped to around 15–20 breaths per minute.[19]

So, what happened in the past 40 years to almost double our respiratory rate? Maybe the same lifestyle changes that have led to a not-dissimilar increase in heart disease, cancer, obesity and dementia over the same period? Or maybe it is the inflammation caused by breathing so fast that has exacerbated those conditions? There are almost certainly correlations either way.

What we can say for sure, however, is that slowing down our breathing, at all times if possible but at least for 20 minutes per day, can have a profound effect on both our everyday health and on our sleep.

And one of the best ways to do that is a technique called Coherent Breathing.

CHAPTER 9

Coherent Breathing

*'Breathe in deeply to bring your
mind home to your body.'*
THICH NHAT HANH

As we have explored, three of the easiest ways to optimize our breathing and therefore sleep better are: inhaling through the nose, increasing lung capacity and breathing much more slowly than usual.

There's a simple breathing technique that encourages all three, while also reducing the symptoms of insomnia, stress and trauma. It's called Coherent Breathing™[1] and it might just change your life.

Search for the Awakened Mind

Stephen Elliott wasn't searching for a breathing technique, he was searching for the brainwave pattern of the awakened mind. And in 1998 the telecommunications scientist and *chi gong* expert managed to find it via a very specific resonant breathing technique that he would later name Coherent Breathing.

Elliott found that breathing at a rate of around five breaths a minute not only created the specific neuro-correlates of the so-called Awakened Mind™[2] state, but also had a profound effect on the autonomic nervous system, bringing about optimal performance in all systems in the body. Breathing at a relaxed rhythm of five breaths per minute, inhaling for six seconds and exhaling for six seconds, creates a state of mind that is deeply relaxed and mindfully alert at the same time. This perfect combination of autonomic balance – relaxation and mental readiness – is quite unique.

Coherent Breathing can be practised by simply counting the length of your breaths, but usually, as it's even better for relaxation, you follow an audio track to keep the specific rhythm. Elliott's most popular Coherent Breathing track is '2 Bells', two Tibetan bells that alternate tones every six seconds. You can find the download link at https://coherentbreathing.com/.

Coherent Breathing can be practised with your eyes open or closed, as a formal meditation practice or informally wherever you are: sitting at your desk, on your morning commute or taking a walk in the park. It's easy to learn, there are no side-effects and the health benefits are huge.

~ *Sleep Notes* ~

When I first heard about the whole five breaths per minute thing, I struggled to believe that something so precise could be applicable for all adults (surely we all have different and unique physiologies?), but all the research backs it up. Five breaths per minute is an almost universal sweet spot for almost all adults.

The Benefits of Coherent Breathing

Breathwork teacher and co-creator of Breath–Body–Mind Dr Richard Brown told me, 'Everything measurable in the lab is optimized by Coherent Breathing, from heart rate variability[3] to brain function to alpha waves[4] – all of it. And it all stays optimized for hours after just 10 minutes of Coherent Breathing.'[5]

His wife, and the other half of Breath–Body–Mind, esteemed professor in psychiatry Dr Patricia Gerbarg, explained to me how it actually works: 'Within a very short time, breathing at five breaths a minute will synchronize the electrical rhythms of the heart, lungs and brain, which is very beneficial and leads to a state in which we are both relaxed and alert. It's unusual to be both relaxed and alert at the same time, but Coherent Breathing creates this sweet spot.'

She continued, 'Most of the medicines that are used to treat anxiety or depression will dampen down the overactivity of the "fight or flight" system, but none of them strengthen the "rest and digest" response. Coherent breathing actually does, though. In fact, it creates a visceral and scientifically verifiable relaxation response within just a few minutes,[6] while also optimizing heart functioning, circulation and nervous system performance.'[7]

Owing to this calming effect on the ANS, Coherent Breathing significantly improves the symptoms of anxiety disorders, PTSD, trauma, stress-related disorders, inflammation, depression and, of course, troubled sleep.

One of the most remarkable benefits is that it may have a similarly detoxifying effect on the brain as deep sleep. This is due to the increase in blood flow that it creates.

Stephen Elliott explained to me exactly how he thought this might work.[8] (This next bit does get quite technical, but it's such a profound proposition in relation to sleep that it's worth exploring in depth.)

Elliott said, 'The average adult body contains five litres of blood, which modern medicine assumes to traverse the body once a minute. Now, you might presume that by slowing down your breath, you slow down that blood flow, but in fact the opposite happens.

'I propose that when we breathe "coherently", the sealed cavity of the chest begins acting as a large slow pump, aiding the heart in facilitating circulation with every coherent breath we take. It does this by generating a wave in the circulatory system that leads to increased pressure differentials that actually increase the rate of blood flow. I hypothesize that when we breathe coherently, the five litres of blood in the body make their way around the circle twice per minute – double the usual speed – owing to this wave created in the circulatory system.'

If this is true, then the increased blood flow would lead to increased circulation of cerebral spinal fluid, which would likewise start to move through the brain more rapidly, flushing out toxins in much the same way as during deep sleep.

This is very exciting possibility, because it means that Coherent Breathing might act as a waking-state method of supplementing the neurological benefits of deep sleep that so many insomniacs are missing out on.

Always Five Breaths per Minute?

This is one of the most frequently asked questions at my workshops, so let's give it a little bit more airtime.

Although breathing anywhere between three and six breaths per minute is good for us, the original protocol defined by Elliott in 2005 specified that 'coherence' (synchronization of the electrical rhythms of the heart and lungs) for most adults occurs at the rate of 5.1 breaths per minute with equal periods of inhalation and exhalation without pause.

Later research confirmed that for most adults, breathing at around five breaths per minute[9] leads to the best level of balance in the nervous system,[10] but anything between three and six breaths per minute still has noticeable benefits.

Breathing more slowly than five breaths per minute won't do you any harm – in fact it can be even more calming and sedating – but Elliott notes that once we reduce breathing frequency to much below four breaths per minute, 'coherence' becomes increasingly distorted, so it seems that five breaths per minute is the best rate for most people.

Having said this, you may well not be *most people*. For the 10 per cent of you reading this who are over six feet tall, your ideal respiratory rate may be a bit slower. It's to do with the greater distance from your extremities to your heart, apparently. So, although it's still advised to learn the practice at five breaths per minute, feel free to transition to four or even three breaths per minute if it feels better for you.[11]

~ *Sleep Notes* ~

Fascinatingly, Professor Luciano Bernadi, a cardiologist at the University of Pavia, Italy, conducted a study that found that reciting the Ave Maria *prayer in Latin slowed respiration to the Coherent Breathing rhythm and that the recitation of certain kundalini yoga mantras did the same,[12] so it seems that five breaths a minute is the speed favoured by both mystics and scientists.*

Exercise:
Coherent Breathing Warm-Up

Going from 15 breaths per minute to five can be quite a radical shift if you haven't done it before, so you might like do some warm-up steps first.

The following warm-up is adapted from *The Healing Power of the Breath* by the stars of our next chapter, Dr Gerbarg and Dr Brown.

~ Sitting in a relaxed posture with your eyes either closed or lightly open, just become aware of how you're breathing. Become aware of breathing in and become aware of breathing out.

~ Whenever you're ready, start following the breathing instructions below, counting silently and slowly in your mind as you do so. Remember this is just a warm-up exercise, so it doesn't need to be very precise, but if in doubt count slower rather than faster.[13]

- Breathing in... two... three.
- Breathing out... two... three.
- Breathing in... two... three.
- Breathing out...two... three

~ Then:

- Breathing in... two... three... four.
- Breathing out... two... three... four.
- Breathing in... two... three... four.
- Breathing out... two... three... four.

~ Repeat the step above, but count a bit more slowly than before.

Remember this is just a warm-up exercise that you might like to try for the first few times before you begin Coherent Breathing.

Exercise: Coherent Breathing

The easiest way to practise Coherent Breathing is to follow an audio track that will help guide your breath into the six-seconds-inhale and six-seconds-exhale rate of five breaths per minute. Most of these audio tracks use a set of repeating chimes or bells with which you can synchronize your breathing rate.

There are loads of different audio tracks and breathing apps available online, but to save you from having to trawl the internet, I've complied links to the Coherent Breathing YouTube channel and the original Coherent Breathing audio tracks created by Elliott for you to stream or download at www.charliemorley.com/wakeuptosleep.

For the expanded Coherent Breathing protocol, be sure to check out Stephen Elliott's book *The New Science of Breath* and his website www. coherentbreathing.com, but for now, here are all the main steps:

~ Sitting comfortably, or lying down if you prefer, eyes closed or lightly open, take three deep relaxing breaths and soften your face, neck and shoulders.

~ Start your chosen Coherent Breathing audio track and simply synchronize your breathing with the track, gently and steadily, with no breath-holding.

~ Breathe in through your nose if possible and don't use any force or pressure. Feel free to slow your breath down gently by dipping in and out of the rhythm for the first couple of minutes until you feel comfortable with the longer breaths.

~ Simply continue to breathe mindfully and gently at the same pace in a relaxed manner. If your mind drifts off, just bring it back to the sensation of your breathing and the sound of the chimes or bells. Allow yourself to relax deeply into the out-breath.

~ Once you are at home with the rhythm, focus on relaxing deeply and releasing tension in your body as you exhale.

~ After your chosen length of time (five, 10 or 20 minutes), gently release your breathing pattern and turn off the audio track. In the silence and stillness that follow, ask yourself: 'How does my body feel now? How does my mind feel right now? What do I notice?'

If you don't have access to an audio track, feel free to do the slow internal count of 'Breathing in... two... three... four...' which we learned in the warm-up exercise above (that will bring you into an approximate five-breaths-per-minute rhythm), but following an audio track is advisable if possible.

Daily Dosage

~ For the first week, aim for 10 or 20 minutes per day in sessions of five or 10 minutes.

~ From the second week onwards, aim for 20 minutes per day, or more if you like.

~ It's recommended that you do 20 minutes of Coherent Breathing a day for 21 days straight to get the optimum benefits.

~ Remember, this is a totally natural way of breathing and you can't overdose on it, so the more you do it, the better. As Elliott says, 'The goal of learning Coherent Breathing is to practise it to the extent that it becomes your normal way of breathing.'[14]

Top Tips for Coherent Breathing

- Be sure to breathe long rather than just slow. The length of the breath is just as important as the speed of it.

- For some people, the first few times they breathe coherently may feel a bit stifling and rigid simply because we so rarely breathe in this perfectly symmetrical way. This feeling will usually pass within a few minutes and isn't anything to worry about. Remember: slow, deep rhythmic breathing is a totally natural way to breathe.

- If you find that you have completed your inhale before the end of the chimes, just pause and then exhale when the next chime sounds.

- You are aiming for your inhale and exhale to be harmoniously balanced, so gently aspire to synchronize with the chimes as much as possible.

- Keeping your eyes either closed or very softly open and your body still has been shown to increase the benefits.

~ Sleep Notes ~

James Nestor, author of Breath: The New Science of a Lost Art, *has a great image to help explain the benefits of slow, deep breathing. He asks us to imagine rowing a boat across a lake. Is taking lots of tiny erratic strokes the most efficient form of rowing? No, slow, rhythmic, long oar strokes is. It's the same with our breathing.*

➤ Field-Tested Feedback

Here's some of the feedback on Coherent Breathing.

Jay, a serving member of the military, told me, 'I've felt a little bit blown away by it, to be honest. For a long time now, I've struggled with sleep for a number of reasons – nightmares, broken sleep, all of that. I really feel that just getting to grips with the Coherent Breathing and slowing down the rate of my breathing have a real physical impact on being able to relax prior to bedtime.'

A military veteran said, 'I'm suffering from a painful physical condition and I've been using Coherent Breathing to calm myself down, and it really helps reduce the pain so I can sleep. It's been great.'

Sarah, a woman working with high levels of stress, told me, 'When I wake up in the night, I do the breathing and my mind comes right down and stops racing. I do the breathing all the time now. It's brilliant.'

For others, it has been the impact on their daytime state of mind that has been most impressive.

One reported: 'I can't say it has changed the way I sleep that much actually, but it has made me much more relaxed during the daytime and much more at ease with my sleep problems.'

Another person found that: 'It's given me an option B in stressful situations, rather than panic, hyperventilate and flip out! Option B is to breathe, relax and realize I'm safe.'

•••

The Yoga Nidra and hypnagogic mindfulness practices that we learned in Part II create deep parasympathetic emphasis, which is great for relaxing deeply and radically lowering stress levels. However, lying down on the floor in a semi-sleep state isn't always practical and we don't always want such deep parasympathetic emphasis anyway, especially if we're driving or at our desk at work. This is why it's great to have Coherent Breathing in our toolbox too, because we *can* do it while we're driving or at our desk at work, as it creates perfect harmony in our ANS: relaxed, but not too relaxed.

In the next chapter we'll explore a set of techniques that build upon this idea of balancing relaxation with mindful awareness by learning a practice that takes Coherent Breathing as its foundation and then adds mindful movement, *chi gong* exercises and a variety of other breathwork techniques to the mix.

Get ready for Breath–Body–Mind…

CHAPTER 10

Breath-Body-Mind

*'There is another way to breathe... a breath of
love that takes you all the way to infinity.'*
RUMI

D r Richard Brown and Dr Pat Gerbarg are a married
couple with more than 100 contributions to medical
research papers between them and they are kind of a big
deal on the trauma integration scene. Pat is a medical doctor
who graduated from Harvard Medical School and is now
assistant clinical professor in psychiatry at New York Medical
College. She is also a herbal medicine expert. Her husband,
Dr Richard Brown, is an associate professor of clinical
psychiatry at Columbia University, with a background in
martial arts, yoga, Zen and *chi gong*. Between them, they have
created a system combining breathwork with meditation and
movements sourced from *chi gong*, yoga and martial arts that
they call Breath-Body-Mind. The core breathwork technique
they use is Coherent Breathing, but crucially they add mindful
movement as a way to further increase its efficacy.

I first met them in 2018 at their home near Woodstock, New York state, as part of my Winston Churchill Memorial Trust research into mindfulness-based approaches to PTSD treatment in veterans.

As I interviewed Dr Brown in their sun-filled garden, he told me, 'Coherent Breathing is a safe, simple method to improve symptoms of stress, trauma and PTSD. But when we combine Coherent Breathing with *chi gong* movements and meditation, we see even better results.'[1]

The Benefits of Breath–Body–Mind

I've found Breath–Body–Mind to be one of the most effective stress and trauma integration practices available.[2] It offers all of the benefits of Coherent Breathing, plus those of mindful movement and bodily awareness, not to mention the subtle energetic and even spiritual benefits of the ancient practice of *chi gong*.

Medical studies have shown that Breath–Body–Mind practices can be used to help treat both psychiatric and physiological conditions. They can help with everything from anxiety and major depressive disorder to inflammatory bowel syndrome and chronic pain.

These practices also activate the social engagement system: the biological network linked to bonding, empathy and affection. Traumatized people desperately need to be able to give and receive affection and love, but they may find it hard to do so, because if their ANS has been severely dysregulated by stress or trauma, it's harder for them to activate their social engagement system. They may find it difficult to be affectionate or accept affection, be touched or touch others, because their ANS is always in 'fight or flight' mode.

Once we regulate the ANS and start to tilt the balance towards parasympathetic emphasis, we will find that showing love and being loved become much easier. And one of the easiest ways to tilt that balance is slow, deep breathing and mindful movement.

With disembodiment (often manifesting as poor physical coordination) and dissociation (feeling disconnected from yourself and the world around you) being common side-effects of trauma, working with the body through mindful movement is a great way to help mitigate these effects.

Dr Gerbarg told me, 'The breathing rhythm and body movements that we use turn down feelings such as fear and anger while turning up our capacity to feel safe, socially engaged and connected to love and compassion. They do this by stimulating the vagus nerves, so increasing the release of the bonding hormone oxytocin while also turning off the "worry centres" in the brain.'[3]

THE SCIENCE OF THE VAGUS NERVES

The vagus nerves start at the brainstem and connect the brain to all the major organs in the body. The vast majority, up to 80 per cent, of their activity is in carrying messages from the body to the brain, so they are the main biological component of the 'body-up' approach to integrating trauma.

Stimulating the vagus nerves releases acetylcholine, which is like a tranquillizer for the nervous system,[4] and oxytocin, which is a bonding chemical often referred to as the 'hugging hormone'. So the vagus nerves not only regulate our organs, but also regulate our mood.

In fact, the vagus nerve network is so strongly linked to the feelings of safety, love and comfort that oxytocin elicits that it has been termed 'the oxytocin superhighway'.

How best to stimulate the vagus nerves and get a hit of both the 'hugging hormone' and deep relaxation? You guessed it: slow, deep breathing.[5]

For Those Who Served

Breath-Body-Mind practices have been taught to active-duty UK and US military and veterans, victims of slavery in Sudan, survivors of the 2010 Haiti earthquake, the genocide in Rwanda and the 9/11 terrorist attacks. I've personally seen iPhone footage from 2011 showing Dr Brown teaching Breath-Body-Mind to a group of 400 South Sudanese refugees who had just been freed from slavery. It's quite moving to watch.

One of the most impressive research studies that Dr Brown has been part of was a randomized controlled trial with 25 Australian Vietnam veterans who had all been classified as 100 per cent clinically disabled because of PTSD for over 30 years. They had received every treatment available to Australian veterans, including high-dose medication as well as group and individual therapy. They all had severe PTSD, with high scores on the PTSD symptom scale. They received an intensive five-day programme of yogic breathing techniques that Dr Brown had modified specifically for veterans and their level of improvement was extraordinary.[6]

One of the veterans, who was suicidal when he came to the programme, told Dr Brown, 'If we'd gotten this when we came back from Vietnam, we wouldn't have lost 30 years of our lives.'

If it works for traumatized veterans and 9/11 survivors, will Breath-Body-Mind be able to help those of us with less severe conditions?

Absolutely. It has been found to be an effective treatment for everyday stress, anxiety and insomnia so it really is a practice that can benefit everyone.

Let's learn how to practise Breath-Body-Mind.

Exercise: Breath-Body-Mind

The Breath-Body-Mind teachings are extensive and thorough, so if you are interested in exploring them in full, please see www.breath-body-mind.com for a list of international workshops both in person and online.

The best way to learn these practices is of course in person with a qualified teacher, but until then let's explore a condensed three-part practice that will have a powerful effect on your general wellbeing as well as your sleep.

Teaching movement through words can often be lost in translation, so you can watch a video demonstrating exactly how to do each part of the following practice at www.charliemorley.com/wakeuptosleep.

Part I: The Ha Breath

Although the predominant practice of Breath-Body-Mind is Coherent Breathing, it often tends to follow a three-part protocol of waking up the body, mindfully synchronizing movement with breath and then, of course, Coherent Breathing.

The Ha Breath is used to wake up our body, raise our energy levels and focus our attention. It also helps release and dispel any feelings that aren't serving us as well as any bodily stress that might be causing anxiety.

Essentially, we draw our arms into our body and then extend them out again while yelling 'Ha!' I know that sounds a bit weird, but it's another great way to ground our awareness in our body while also helping to release tension from our body, which can actually make the Coherent Breathing easier to do.

The Ha Breath is also a great way to counteract dissociation (one of the key features of PTSD and trauma), because it not only grounds our awareness into our body, but also lets us feel a sense of 'Here is my body. This is where my body ends. This is where my body begins. I am embodied.'

NB: The Ha Breath should not be done by people with high blood pressure, seizure disorder or bipolar disorder, or who are pregnant or have had recent surgery. The forceful and rapid exhalation can transiently elevate blood pressure, which may be problematic for members of the aforementioned groups. The Ha Breath and all of the following practices can be done seated as well as standing.

How do you do it?

~ Standing with your feet shoulder-width apart, raise both your arms to chest height as if you are carrying a tray of drinks on your forearms. Inhale through your nose as you bend and draw your elbows back with your palms facing upwards in light fists.

~ Exhale forcefully through your mouth with the sound '*Ha!*' while extending your arms forward and turning your palms down (like shaking water off your fingertips).

~ Repeat this 15 times.

~ Relax and pause for about 15 seconds as you stand with your arms by your sides, closing your eyes or gazing downwards.

~ Then, if you like, you can repeat the previous steps three times (a maximum of three sets of 15 Ha Breaths in total).

Part II: 4-4 Arm Circles

Now that your body has woken up and been energized, you can move on to the mindful movement in synchronization with your breath. The 4-4 arm circles practice is based on a *chi gong* sequence in which movements are synchronized with a slow four-count breathing rhythm.

The breathing rate for this exercise can be maintained by doing a slow internal count of four or by using your preferred Coherent Breathing audio track. Either is fine.

~ Stand with your feet beneath your hips and your hands resting below your navel, palms up, with your fingertips lightly touching.

~ As you inhale to a count of four (or follow a Coherent Breathing audio track), raise your hands and gradually turn your palms outwards and upwards as you raise your arms up above your head with your palms facing the sky.

~ As you exhale to a count of four (or follow a Coherent Breathing audio track), make a wide circle with your hands, reaching out towards the horizon on either side all the way down to the starting position.

~ Repeat this process 8–16 times.

~ Stand with your feet shoulder-width apart, arms relaxed at your sides, and go inwards, check in and release this part of the practice.

If you are going to do this exercise using your own count rather than the audio track, it should be like this:

~ Breathe in… two… three… four… (as you raise your hands upwards until your palms are facing the sky).

~ Then breathe out… two… three… four… (as you make a big circle lowering your hands down to the starting position).

Part III: Coherent Breathing

Now that your breath has been both synchronized with your body and slowed down to within the Coherent Breathing range, you can move to a seated or lying position and continue with the standard Coherent Breathing practice that you learned previously.

~   Sit comfortably or lie down.

~   Play your chosen Coherent Breathing audio track.

~   Follow the instructions from the previous chapter (*see p.117*).

~   After your chosen length of time (five, 10 or 20 minutes), gently release the breathing pattern, turn off the audio track and check in with your body and mind: how do you feel after the practice?

Daily Dosage

One 20-minute session a day for ordinary stress reduction.

If you are working with depression, anxiety or PTSD, 40 minutes a day (two 20-minute sessions if possible).

As the Ha Breath and 4-4 arm circles only take five minutes or so, Coherent Breathing will make up the majority of your practice.

Resistance Breathing and Belly Breathing

There are two additional ways that many people find helpful to maximize the effects of Breath–Body–Mind teaching.

Resistance Breathing

Resistance breathing is a way to make the slow, deep breathing even more beneficial. There are lots of ways to practise it, but essentially it's about creating some slight resistance as you exhale.

The two recommended resistance breathing techniques are:

- 'The pursed lips exhale' in which you purse your lips as if about to whistle and then exhale through them. The inhale remains through the nose.

- The yogic Ujjayi ocean breath, sometimes called 'the Darth Vader breath', in which you exhale with an audible sound similar to either the ocean or (spoiler alert) Luke Skywalker's dad.

Belly Breathing

Belly breathing, otherwise known as diaphragmatic breathing, is when you inhale down into your belly, which will naturally expand, allowing for a longer, deeper breath. Breathing into your belly is much more natural than breathing only into your chest and has a whole host of benefits, including increased stress reduction and parasympathetic activation.

~ Sleep Notes ~

Remember, it all comes down to this: the brain listens to the lungs above all else, and so slow, deep rhythmic breathing is one of the most direct ways to tell the brain: 'All is well. We are safe. Nothing to run from and nothing to fight. Time to relax, stand down and feel peaceful.'

➤ Field-Tested Feedback

Many people find that the added layer of mindful movement and embodiment that Breath–Body–Mind offers leads to even deeper benefits than Coherent Breathing alone. When I taught it to a group containing many people with PTSD, the feedback included: 'It brought together the other learning and techniques in a holistic way – all the stuff about the body needing to be engaged. It all made sense.'

For some, it was their favourite technique of the six-week course: 'I find practising Coherent Breathing with arm movements very helpful. I feel more peaceful and less anxious during the day and sleep more deeply at night with these practices.'

Although lots of people find that it helps with their sleep, just as many of the testimonials about Breath–Body–Mind focus on its impact on the waking state, for example: 'Breath–Body–Mind was my biggest learning of the course and I felt the most positive change in my daily life from it.'

And simply: 'When I started doing Breath–Body–Mind for 20 mins every day, my panic attacks stopped.'

•••

In Chapter 13 we'll explore three breathwork techniques especially designed for people working with nightmares or night terrors. For now, though, concentrate on creating a daily practice of at least 20 minutes of either Coherent Breathing or Breath–Body–Mind or both.

Part III Checklist ✓

✓ Be sure to practise at least 20 minutes of either Coherent Breathing and/or Breath-Body-Mind every day, or twice a day if possible for those working with PTSD or trauma. Even one or two sessions a week can still make a big impact, so just as with Yoga Nidra, something is better than nothing.

✓ Keep up the regular Yoga Nidra/hypnagogic mindfulness practice too. If you choose to do your Coherent Breathing lying down, they may well start to meld into each other. That's fine. The main thing is to give yourself at least half an hour of deep rest and relaxation practice every day.

✓ Regular entries into your Nocturnal Journal are a must, especially now, as many people find that Coherent Breathing noticeably affects the quality and duration of their sleep.

✓ Don't forget to breathe slowly and through your nose in order to expand your lungs and live longer.

PART IV

NIGHTMARE INTEGRATION

'Perhaps everything that frightens us is, in its deepest essence, something helpless that wants our love... You must realize that something is happening to you, that life has not forgotten you, that it holds you in its hand and will not let you fall.'

RAINER MARIA RILKE, *LETTERS TO A YOUNG POET*

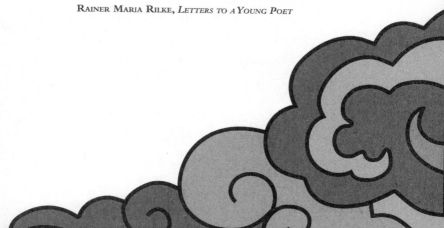

Over the past 13 years I've worked with hundreds of nightmare sufferers, including victims of childhood abuse, survivors of terrorist attacks and of course armed forces veterans and serving military personnel.

What I've noticed is that for many people, the deepest healing has come not from trying to 'get rid' of their nightmares as much as from a shift of perspective concerning what nightmares are actually trying to do.

Many of us, quite understandably, pathologize our nightmares and view them as a 'sign of a broken mind', but this simply isn't true. Nightmares are a *call to action* from the unconscious mind, a sign of healing, not of failure. Once we understand that, a new road to transformation opens up to us.

Whether you are currently working with nightmares or not, if you can heed the healing call to face and embrace them, you may well find that they are like dragons guarding a pot of gold. Crucially though, our aim is not to slay the dragon but to befriend it.

CHAPTER 11

Nightmares

'The cave you fear to enter holds the treasure you seek.'
JOSEPH CAMPBELL

As I mentioned in the introduction, I was 17 when I experienced my first trauma nightmare. After taking a misguidedly large dose of ketamine while tripping on a misguidedly large dose of LSD, I had a full-on tunnel of light, entering the void, near-death experience.

Although nowadays I might respond to such an episode in a very different way, as a teenager it totally overwhelmed my ability to cope, and within days the nightmares and night terrors began. They recurred weekly for the next few months,[1] then started coming at other times too, as did the flashbacks and panic attacks that had me hiding in the toilet cubicles at school. At night I would try to stay awake, too scared to sleep, but eventually sleep would come, and with it the nightmares and the terror that would crush me. Looking back on it now, it seems such an obvious case of trauma and PTSD, but at the time I'm not sure if I even knew what that meant. All I knew was that I had 'fucked up my brain'.

If only I'd known then what I know now – that what I was going through was a totally normal response to trauma and part of a totally natural healing process. Normal and natural. If only I'd known.

In the end, too scared of diagnosis to seek medical help, I took matters into my own hands and, after months of trying, managed to use lucid dreaming to cure the nightmares. I became lucidly aware within the nightmare and intentionally turned towards the source of my fear. By finally facing the nightmare consciously, the trauma that was creating it was spontaneously integrated. The nightmares never came back. In fact, it was the visceral and undeniable success of that lucid dream healing that started me off down the road that would eventually, 20 years later, lead to this book.

In the following chapters we're going to learn the techniques that I used to cure those nightmares, plus loads more too, but before that, let's take a deep dive into what nightmares actually are.

A Nightmare Defined

The American Academy of Sleep Medicine defines nightmares as 'vivid and disturbing dreams typically involving threats to survival, which evoke emotions of anxiety, fear or terror' in the sleeping subject. They are typically scenarios in which we are either fighting off or fleeing from terrifying dream characters and situations or replaying emotional trauma caused by a real-life event. Nightmares affect an estimated 90 per cent of those who have experienced trauma[2] and are a totally normal response that actually aids the healing process. Nightmares aren't always linked to trauma, though, and can occur for a variety of reasons, including mental and physical health challenges, as a side-effect of the drugs used to treat those challenges, and often, just like anxiety dreams, as fire drills for possible future dangers.

Nightmares are often so stimulatingly scary that they not only leave a somatic resonance in our body, but often actually interrupt our usual REM cycle and wake us up. Every time we wake from a nightmare, however, the unintegrated emotional energy that led to the nightmare remains unintegrated. That's why our nightmares tend to recur: not because our mind is torturing us, but because it is trying to finish an internal therapy session that got cut short.

Nightmares aren't punishment for what we've done, they aren't a sign of moral failure, they aren't proof of a broken mind. They are the product of an intelligent emotional regulation mechanism that actually helps to keep us sane.

We need to at least reframe and at most totally revolutionize our view of them.

Reframing Nightmares

I first wrote about the following three 'reframes' in my 2017 book about Shadow integration, *Dreaming Through Darkness*.

Since then, both the arguments for them and the science supporting them have become much stronger.

The science is clear: most of the time, nightmares are good for our mental health. They help us heal, they update our evolutionary survival mechanisms and they draw our attention to emotional wounds that we may be blindsided by while awake.

A Dream That Is Shouting

Nightmares don't mean to hurt us; they mean to grab our attention. A nightmare is simply a dream that is shouting. It is shouting, 'Hey, look at this! Deal with this fear! This trauma needs attention!'

Dr Justin Havens, a psychological therapist who conducted his PhD research into the PTSD nightmares of veterans, agrees, saying, 'When bad things happen, we are *supposed* to dream about them, because the nightmare is highlighting a problematic aspect such as unresolved emotional distress that needs to be integrated.'[3]

Just as physical pain is used by our brain to tell us to attend to a wounded part of our body, so nightmares are used by our unconscious mind to make us attend to a wounded part of our psyche. The nightmare is not shouting in order to scare us but to help us. And so, if we want to reduce the frequency of our nightmares, we need to do everything we can to tell our unconscious mind, 'Okay, okay! I'm listening. No need to shout!'

This can be done by writing our nightmares down, drawing pictures of them or discussing them with a therapist or trusted friend. Essentially, we want to do everything we can to show the unconscious mind that we hear it loud and clear.

This is the opposite of the New Age delusion that claims that to write a nightmare down or to recount it out loud might serve to 'manifest it into reality'. This kind of spiritual bypassing is not only complete bullshit, but may also be a dangerous slide into denial and the depression that often results from it. In fact, through the act of bearing witness to a nightmare, we can release the underlying emotional charge or trauma that was creating it and allow it to be integrated into our psycho-physical system.

Essentially, if we are willing to face rather than reject our nightmares, we can foster a shift of perspective that tells them: 'I hear you. I understand that you're an expression of my own mind that is shouting for attention.' And upon receiving that message, the dreaming mind won't feel the need to shout so loudly in future.

This new perspective may spill over into our waking life, too, and we may start to view nightmarish situations with new eyes and a new appreciation of the potential for healing that they offer.

THE SCIENCE OF NIGHTMARE RESOLUTION

Scientific research indicates that our dreams are a litmus test for trauma integration. Once a trauma has been integrated, whether in the dream state or waking state, our dreams will reflect this.

The brilliant young sleep scientist Dr Michelle Carr says, 'It seems that because recurrent nightmares are revealing some unresolved conflict, once the successful integration has occurred, the nightmare is no longer necessary and will stop occurring.'[4]

She comments that the cessation of a recurrent nightmare is a sign that the trauma has been confronted and adaptively integrated in the psyche, which, unsurprisingly, is associated with improved waking-state wellbeing.[5]

Dr Carr also mentions how having a resolution dream in which the nightmare finally ends differently – the fear is faced or the attacker is befriended, for example – often precedes the cessation of nightmares. She suggests that remembering and keeping track of our dreams is not only a good way to notice this, but also helpful in aiding this process.[6] Another good reason to write down our dreams in our Nocturnal Journal.

~ Sleep Notes ~

My Buddhist teacher Lama Yeshe Rinpoche had nightmares for years after his traumatic escape from Tibet in the 1960s. He knew the trauma was integrated when his usual nightmare was replaced by a resolution dream in which Chinese leader Mao Zedong was helping him to stack shelves in a dream grocery store that he owned. After that, his nightmares stopped.

A Sign of a Healing Mind

Our mind uses nightmares to treat and heal its wounds. If we cut our arm, our body bleeds and then sends coagulates and white blood cells to form a protective layer over the wound to prevent any further damage. This allows the healing process to continue below the surface. If this didn't happen, we might end up with sepsis or gangrene from every minor wound.

A nightmare works in a similar way: it's a manifestation of the healing process used by the mind to regulate emotion and integrate traumatic experiences. Just like a scab, it can be itchy and unsightly and we might try to hide it from others, and yet it's vital to the healing process. Also, just as if we keep picking at a scab it can lead to further bleeding, if we pick at or dwell on our nightmares too much, this can slow up the healing process.

It's all about balance. We need to acknowledge and welcome our nightmares by writing them down and being willing to witness and accept them, but we also need to make sure that we don't become overly identified with them.

Of course, I'm not suggesting that we *have* to have nightmares in order to heal, but if trauma remains unwitnessed and thus unintegrated, our mind's natural self-healing mechanism will take things into its own hands.

For healing to occur, our mind and body have to process and release the trauma. This can happen in one of three main ways:

- Through the conscious mind (via talking therapy or mindfulness and insight training, for example).

- Through the body (via the breath, somatic release or mindful movement, for example).

- Through the unconscious mind (via dreams, nightmares and imaginal practices).

Quite understandably, many people are unwilling to intentionally bear witness to their past traumas through either their conscious mind or their body, and so the trauma has no other option but to express itself through nightmares.

Although unpleasant, this isn't actually a bad option because REM sleep is custom-built for integrating trauma.

Studies led by the brilliant Dr Rosalind Cartwright at Rush University in Chicago looking at the effects of depression caused by trauma showed that 'only patients who were expressly dreaming about the painful experiences' around the time of them actually happening became clinically free of their depression. Those who were dreaming, but not actually dreaming about their emotionally painful or traumatic experiences, showed no such improvement. Healing was predicated on 'dreaming about the emotional themes and sentiments of the waking state trauma'.[7]

I was so excited when I first came across this research, because it scientifically proved that dreaming about the painful experiences actually *hastened* the healing process and helped to reduce long-term depression, a fact that will bring relief to many people working with nightmares.

Professor Matthew Walker had long theorized that REM was needed in order to heal from emotional wounds, but in 2011 he conducted a study that proved his theory neurobiologically.[8] Using EEG and MRI brain scans, he concluded that REM dreaming sleep actually changed the nervous system, leading to a measurable decrease in the emotional intensity of previous traumatic experiences.

Both of these studies show beyond doubt that dreaming about our fears, unpleasant experiences and heartbreak is not only good for us, but often actually a prerequisite for healing.

Nightmares as an Evolutionary Tool

Whereas our first two reframes explain how nightmares help to integrate past traumas, our third one explains how they may be used to help us survive future ones too.

One of the key reasons that we came to be top predators on the planet was our ability to dream, and thus explore future actions. But more specifically, it was our ability to have nightmares.

Professor Antti Revonsuo, a Finnish scientist who created the threat simulation theory of dreaming, believes that REM dreaming is 'an ancient biological defence mechanism, evolutionarily selected for its capacity to repeatedly simulate threatening events'.[9] We have scary dreams so that we are better placed to survive scary situations in waking life.

Imagine two prehistoric women sharing a cave. One of them regularly has nightmares about sabre-toothed tigers and how to fight them, run from them or hide from them, while the other one has peaceful dreams about walking around the savannah.

If they were to meet a sabre-toothed tiger in waking life, which would be better placed to survive and pass on her genes? The one who had been rehearsing how to survive in her dreams, of course.

Professor Revonsuo concludes, 'Nightmares force us to go through simulated threatening events so that in the waking world we are more prepared to survive them.'[10] Proof again that, just like anxiety dreams, nightmares can actually be good for us.

Most of the time, anyway...

PTSD Dreaming

As we've discussed, nightmares are a rehearsal space for daytime threats and a safe place for traumas to be highlighted and healed, but unfortunately the effects of PTSD on the brain can disrupt all that.

It's all down to elevated levels of stress hormones. There is a stress chemical called noradrenaline (also known as norepinephrine) that is almost always present in the brain in low amounts, but completely absent during REM sleep. This is so that when we dream about traumatic experiences, we can process the upsetting memories in a 'safe space' free from stress hormones.

Sleep scientist Dr Els van der Helm explains that 'During REM sleep, painful memories are being reactivated and integrated, but this all happens in a state where stress neurochemicals are beneficially suppressed.'[11]

However, in people with PTSD, the level of noradrenaline in their brain is markedly higher at all times, including when they dream, meaning that when they do so, they are dreaming in a space that has not been 'made safe'. These high levels of noradrenaline during REM *prevent* the healing quality of the nightmares that occur within it. And so, for people with PTSD, nightmares may be more like retraumatizing flashbacks than healing therapeutic interventions.

This may also explain why nightmares recur so frequently in those with PTSD. Being unable to use REM sleep to integrate the traumatic memories as per usual, the brain will attempt the integration process over and over again, getting stuck on a loop like a broken record.

But here's the good news: if we can reduce the level of noradrenaline in our brain, we can create conditions that allow the natural healing process of REM dreaming to occur and the needle on the record to be lifted.

This can be done in two main ways: either chemically, with noradrenaline-reducing medication such as Prazosin, which is already being offered to treat PTSD symptoms, or naturally, through exactly the same kind of stress-reducing slow breathing, deep relaxation and mindfulness practices that we have learned so far.

➤ Field-Tested Feedback

Many people find that just learning about these new perspectives on nightmares has a big impact on reducing the fear they create.

One workshop participant said: 'It seems that nightmares are the beginning of a healing process and should be approached and embraced, rather than be ignored or fled from. That's a big shift for me.'

Another commented: 'Just understanding how nightmares work and that they are normal for people with PTSD was so helpful for me.'

•••

In Chapters 13 and 15 we are going learn some of the most effective techniques for integrating nightmares, but before that, let's explore and destigmatize two other night-time manifestations of stress and trauma: night terrors and sleep paralysis.

CHAPTER 12

Night Terrors and Sleep Paralysis

'Even in the terrors of the night, there is a
tendency toward grace that does not fail us.'
ROBERT GOOLRICK, AUTHOR OF
THE END OF THE WORLD AS WE KNOW IT

Nightmares happen while we're asleep, but night terrors and sleep paralysis occur in a liminal hinterland in which the boundaries between sleep and waking blur. They are both pretty common for people working with trauma, PTSD or high levels of stress and anxiety, but, just like nightmares, once you know how they work, they become much less scary.

Night Terrors

A night terror is quite different from a nightmare. Whereas nightmares usually occur in REM dreaming sleep, night terrors aren't actually linked with dreaming at all and are more akin to night-time panic attacks.

Usually occurring in the first three or four hours of sleep (when the longer deep-sleep periods occur), they tend to happen in the hypnopompic transition from deep sleep to waking.

During a night terror, we may sit bolt upright in bed, eyes open, heart pounding, maybe even screaming, and be unable to be roused from this state for several minutes. Night terrors can overlap with a form of sleepwalking too, and we might run from our bed to try to escape the unseen threat.

These episodes of extreme panic and unadulterated fear usually have none of the scary narrative or visuals of a nightmare and if you ask the person to explain what was so terrifying, they will often have no answer to give[1] or just describe a feeling of doom or of needing to escape something.

Due to the saving grace of that amnesia, plus the fact that the mind is still saturated in the relaxing delta brainwaves of deep sleep, afterwards people often just lie back down and go to sleep, often not even remembering the episode when they wake in the morning.

The late, great sleep researcher Dr William Dement theorized that during a night terror we might not be experiencing fear at all, because it is the body that is expressing fright rather than the mind. This view on night terrors is particularly interesting in relation to our body-based approach to trauma, because it seems to suggest that once the body has discharged the traumatic stressors, sleep can proceed naturally.

What Causes a Night Terror?

Night terrors most frequently affect children between three and 12 years old and have a strong genetic element, with around 80 per cent of those children having a family history of them.[2]

For adults, night terrors can be caused by short-term conditions such as fever, sleep deprivation, jet lag or drug use, but are most commonly associated with psychological challenges, such as trauma, high levels of stress, depression, anxiety or bipolar disorder.

There is also a link between night terrors and respiratory issues such as sleep apnoea, which is why techniques like Coherent Breathing seem to work so well for night terrors: they not only calm the out-of-kilter ANS, but also strengthen the respiratory system.

How can we prevent night terrors? Rebalance the ANS through slow breathing, calm the mind through mindfulness practices and reduce stress levels through deep relaxation. In the next chapter there is a practice called Circle of Protectors, which people find especially helpful for working with both nightmares and night terrors.

Sleep Paralysis

Sleep paralysis is the experience of waking up with the inability to move, sometimes accompanied by feelings of pressure on the chest, as if being held down, feelings of fear and dread, and often visual and auditory hallucinations too. For most people, this is a terrifying experience, as the hallucinatory images and sounds may lead them to believe that demons are trying to possess them or that there are dark forces in the room.

Sleep paralysis most commonly occurs during the hypnopompic state, but sometimes during the hypnagogic too. Although it may seem to go on for hours, it rarely lasts for more than a couple of minutes and is actually quite a common occurrence.

THE SCIENCE OF SLEEP PARALYSIS

Sleep paralysis is caused by one of the three REM sleep systems, muscular paralysis, staying engaged when the other two, sensory blockade and cortical activation, have been disengaged, meaning that while our brain has partially woken up and our senses are taking in partial sensory input, our physical body cannot move.

Due to our brain's momentary engagement in both the dream state and waking state, hallucinatory images may be superimposed over our normal field of vision, and there are often loud audio hallucinations too. The fear that this altered state generates can also lead to hyperventilation, and in turn a feeling of weight on our chest. This often goes together with hypnagogic hallucinations: aural and visual dream aspects superimposed over the waking world.

Now add to the mix the fact that sleep paralysis is often accompanied by a form of hyperacusis, a condition in which sounds become amplified and distorted, and we can see why in earlier times possession by a demon often seemed to be the best explanation.

Sleep paralysis has been referenced throughout history and across all cultures. From the Japanese *kanashibari*, 'fastened in metal', to the Zimbabwean *madzikirira*, 'strongly pressed down by a witch', to the incubus/succubus myths of the West, the phenomenon of waking up from sleep paralysed by terror has been universally mythologized. The subjective symptoms seem to be pretty universal too.

Thankfully, we now know that sleep paralysis is a neurologically explained phenomenon, which helps to put the demonic myths of the past to bed.

~ *Sleep Notes* ~

Confusingly, sleep paralysis can also occur within a 'false awakening': a dream in which we dream that we have woken up, but in fact we're still asleep. So, although it feels as though your eyes are open and you are witnessing hallucinations superimposed over your bedroom, you may well be simply dreaming that your eyes are open and that you are witnessing those hallucinations.

Links to Trauma

My friend Ryan Hurd is a psychology lecturer at JFK University, California, and the author of *Sleep Paralysis: A Guide to Hypnagogic Visions and Visitors of the Night*. When we spoke over Zoom in early 2021, he confirmed that occasional sleep paralysis could be caused by a variety of reasons, including a disrupted sleep schedule or sleep apnoea, as well as stress, drug use, or simply major life change. But for people working with panic disorders, trauma or PTSD, the frequency skyrockets. A 2018 analysis of 42 scientific studies[3] into sleep paralysis found that those who had been diagnosed with PTSD showed significantly higher rates across multiple studies.

Ryan told me, 'For those who have encountered trauma, especially those who have suffered from childhood sexual abuse, sleep paralysis is a very common symptom.'[4]

He explained that bad sleep and high anxiety created the perfect storm for sleep paralysis[5] and so people struggling with stress, anxiety or trauma in addition to poor sleep were much more likely to experience it.

Integrating Sleep Paralysis

In the long run, the best way to prevent sleep paralysis from happening is to lower the stress and anxiety levels that are most likely to be triggering it, while also improving the poor sleep patterns that exacerbate it. So, practices like mindfulness, breathwork and deep relaxation will definitely help. But what about when we are actually experiencing it?

The best course of action then is to activate the parasympathetic nervous system through the breath. This will reduce the 'fight or flight' fear response that is both causing and concretizing the sleep paralysis.

As Ryan said, 'It's so important to try to relax and breathe normally rather than maintaining the shallow gasping breaths that the fear of the situation so often leads to. Once we take control of our breath, we take control of our fear response.'[6]

I used to get sleep paralysis a lot and my personal tip is to engage, or even just imagine engaging, a long, extended out-breath, either through your nose or, if possible, your front teeth, making a sound similar to letting air out of a tyre. This creates a relaxation of the respiratory system and an activation of the parasympathetic response that will help to disengage the paralysis.

Another option is to stay with the experience but transform its content. Sleep paralysis hallucinations are sourced from *within our own mind* and so they reflect the internal environment of our mind, which, during sleep paralysis, is usually one of total fear. For some, that fear might create visions of ghosts or aliens, but for those suffering from trauma, it might recreate visions of the traumatic experiences. But if we can change that internal mental environment from one of fear to one of love, we may very well see those hallucinated demons turn into angels before our very eyes. 'Just think happy thoughts' is an oversimplification, but if we can create an internal environment of love and safety then this will directly impact the experience.

This is easier said than done of course, but it is totally possible and explains why so many people break out of sleep paralysis when they pray: the act of prayer changes the internal environment of their mind from fear to love.

~ *Sleep Notes* ~

Sleep paralysis gives us one foot in the waking state and one foot in the dream state, which can be ideal for entering a lucid dream. So, if you're feeling confident, you can intentionally stay with it, knowing that you are safe to re-enter the dream from whence you came, but lucidly this time. What might you do then? For some ideas, see Chapter 15.

Sleep paralysis can make people think they're going crazy and so they suffer in shamed silence, but it isn't a sign of madness and it doesn't have to be dreaded. Most probably you haven't been possessed by demons, you aren't going mad and there aren't any dark forces in your bedroom. All that is happening is that your brain has woken up before your body has, due to an imbalance in your ANS – something that you can absolutely put right. Then you can sleep peacefully again.

CHAPTER 13

Nightmare Integration Exercises

'Go to places that scare you in order to
discover the Buddha within yourself.'
MACHIG LABDRÖN, ELEVENTH-CENTURY TIBETAN YOGINI

Whether you're suffering from nightmares, night terrors or sleep paralysis, all the practices we've mentioned so far, especially Yoga Nidra and Coherent Breathing, will help to integrate and lessen the effects. But I also want to offer you a set of techniques specifically designed to help those of you currently working with nightmares.

The following techniques have been successfully used by people with high levels of PTSD and trauma, as well as those with none, so they are all safe to use and all very effective.

Exercise: Circle of Protectors

This exercise was inspired by an ancient practice within the Tibetan indigenous lineage of Bön and it's particularly helpful for anyone working with nightmares, night terrors or pre-sleep anxiety. It's always one of the favourite techniques when I work with groups who are experiencing PTSD trauma nightmares in particular.

The original Tibetan teachings say that if you are feeling scared or anxious before you sleep, you should turn your sleeping area into a sacred protected space by imagining that you are surrounded by powerful protectors, enlightened beings and Dakinis (female embodiments of awakening), who remain 'like mothers watching over a child or guardians surrounding a king or queen'.[1]

Those of us not so connected to Tibetan notions of enlightened beings can visualize anyone or anything who offers us a feeling of love, safety, allegiance and protection. Our protectors can be living or dead, real or unreal, known or unknown. They can be superheroes or buddhas, mythical warriors or religious symbols, ancestors or planets. Some people fall asleep imagining themselves surrounded by huge buffalos, Jesus Christ, MMA fighters and the wizard Gandalf, all of whom stand guard while they sleep.

Personally, I might imagine my Buddhist teacher Lama Yeshe Rinpoche and the eighth-century Tantric master Padamsambhava alongside a huge shamanic power animal like a garuda and the blazing sun in each of the four cardinal directions, and then I might fill the gaps with fire, crystals, mountains and galaxies. There are no rules for this – you can't get it wrong, so don't limit yourself. Be creative.

The Buddhist teachings say that the mind with which we fall asleep flavours the whole night that follows, so if we can fall asleep with a feeling of protection and safety, our sleep and dreams will follow suit. So feel free to do this practice even if you're not currently working with nightmares, as it can help you fall asleep feeling relaxed and calm, which will then allow you to sleep better too.

You can do this practice by following the guided audio meditation track that I've made at www.charliemorley.com/wakeuptosleep or you can guide yourself through the steps below.

~ Decide which protectors you're going to invoke. Lying in bed before sleep, close your eyes and allow yourself to relax into the shallows of the hypnagogic.

~ Imagine your first protector standing or sitting near your head. You don't have to see them clearly, just know that they're there, watching over you, protecting you, holding you in their love.

~ Next, imagine your second protector sitting or standing by your feet. Your second protector is watching over you with love. Feel the power of their protection.

~ Now, imagine your third protector on your left-hand side. Feel their love, their safety beaming down to you. You now have protectors by your head, your feet and your left-hand side. You don't have to see them clearly, just know that they're there.

~ And now imagine your fourth protector sitting or standing by your right-hand side, watching over you and exuding a feeling of safety, of love.

~ Take a moment to feel the love, the safety and the protection your protectors are offering you. You're surrounded by protection. You're surrounded by love.

~ And finally, fill in the gaps between the protectors. Again, you could do this with people or animals or balls of light, crystals, fire, weapons, stars, galaxies, fairy lights… Whatever you choose, fill in the gaps between each of the four primary protectors, completing your circle of protectors.

Hold that visualization for as long as you can, then let it fade, let it slip from your mind's eye as you drift through the hypnagogic state and into sleep, knowing you are protected.

Daily Dosage

Every night if you like, or as and when required. You can even do it in the waking state if you are feeling overwhelmed or anxious.

~ Sleep Notes ~

At an ultimate level, this exercise is, however, superfluous. Partly because there is nothing in your mind that you need to be protected from and partly because your protectors are with you at all times anyway. They are within you and have never left your side, not once. In fact, this exercise doesn't as much call them in as open your eyes to see that they're already there.

➤ Field-Tested Feedback

My friend Donna Dee is a UK garage DJ. She did a six-week 'Mindfulness of Dream & Sleep' course with me and out of all the practices, she found that Circle of Protectors was the real breakthrough for her. She told me:

I've always had trouble sleeping. I just feel uneasy and unsafe as I fall asleep, and I have nightmares too.

I've tried pretty much everything, but nothing worked until I tried Circle of Protectors. I imagine all these Buddhist deities around me and I can really feel their energy. Most of the time I don't actually get to the end of it, because I feel so relaxed that I fall asleep! It's one of the most useful practices I've ever come across, but I don't actually use it anymore because I don't need to: the fear's gone. The practice shifted something.

A woman called Stella, who was on the same course, found the practice had a similarly powerful effect:

Bed has never felt like a safe or relaxing place for me, as I was sexually abused by my father, and I also spent a lot of time lying awake at night listening out to hear if he was attacking my mother, so it's deeply embedded in my body to stay alert in bed, to not let go into sleep, in case something happens.

The Circle of Protectors feels like the missing piece for me. I followed your guided instructions on YouTube last night and it felt so good to allow all that safety in. My husband was at my head, Jesus was at my feet, a grassy meadow was to my left and sun rays were to my right. I felt worthy of safety and protection. I felt like a queen. I fell asleep so easily. I didn't need to stay on guard, as I usually do. This is huge for me.

Exercise: The 4,7,8 Breath

It's 4 a.m. and you've just woken from a nightmare. You're feeling shaken and can't get back to sleep. Or maybe you've been in bed for hours, lying awake because you're just too wired to sleep? You need the 4,7,8 Breath: inhaling for a count of four, holding your breath for a count of seven and exhaling for a count of eight.

Whereas the Coherent Breathing five-breaths-per minute rhythm is great at creating perfect balance in the ANS, extending the out-breath (in this case, doubling it) will shift the emphasis towards the parasympathetic.

Medical studies have shown that when the out-breath is longer than the in-breath, there is greater stimulation of the 'rest and digest' system, leading to an even more calming and physically relaxing response than equal breath length.[2]

In some ways, even more important than the extended exhale is the seven-count breath hold, as it helps to gently increase carbon dioxide levels, which helps to dilate blood vessels throughout the body. As a result, blood pressure is lowered and a deeper state of relaxation can be reached.

For many people, Coherent Breathing is more than enough to remove the stressors that prevent sleep, but if you ever need a little more parasympathetic drive, then try the 4,7,8 Breath. Great for before bed, not so great for operating heavy machinery!

Dr Andy Weil, founder of the Arizona Center for Integrative Medicine, has conducted a lot of research into its effects. He says, 'This is a great way to help you fall asleep. Or if you wake up in the middle of the night and can't get back to sleep, this technique will help you fall asleep right away.'[3]

The 4,7,8 Breath is a natural tranquilliser for the nervous system. But unlike tranquillizing drugs, which often lose their power over time, this exercise gains in power with repetition and practice.

NB: The seven-count breath hold should not be done by those who are pregnant or those with severe respiratory conditions.

~ Sitting comfortably, ready for sleep, place your tongue behind your upper front teeth and exhale completely and audibly through your mouth.

~ Now close your mouth and inhale through your nose for a count of four.

~ Hold your breath for a count of seven.

~ Release your breath through your mouth audibly for a count of eight.

Repeat this process four times for the first few times you do it, then increase the repetitions as many times as you like up to 12 times in a row.

Daily Dosage

As and when required – during the day, before bed, in the middle of the night. This is a great addition to your relaxation toolbox.

~ Sleep Notes ~

The 4,7,8 Breath isn't a new invention, it's a form of pranayama *from the ancient yogic system of India. Prana means 'life-force', often translated as 'breath', and* yama *means 'control' or 'restraint', so* pranayama *can be translated as 'breath control'. Its true meaning is much more nuanced, though, as* pranayama *is actually more about allowing the life-force to flow rather than controlling it.*

➤ Field-Tested Feedback

I taught the 4,7,8 Breath to an Italian lady named Adette, who was attending a lucid dreaming retreat I was running in Venice. She told me it totally changed the way she slept. 'It made me feel safer and more relaxed. It was as if I'd taken a relaxation pill! I slept better the first night I used it, so I started using it every night after that. And even during the daytime, too, if I felt stressed. And if I wake up in the night now, I do a few rounds of the breathing and soon fall back asleep.'

•••

Exercise: Nightmare Rescripting

Nightmare Rescripting is a creative writing and drawing exercise in which we 'download' our nightmare onto the page through words and imagery, and then, most importantly, consciously change the ending or outcome.

The version that I teach draws its inspiration from Dr Justin Havens' Planned Dream Intervention (PDI) as well as Dr Deidre Barrett's work at Harvard on dream incubation.

Dr Havens believes that waking ourselves from a nightmare prevents the dream content from being fully integrated, but if we can create an alternate ending to our recurring nightmare while we are awake – the car doesn't crash or we are saved from the attack, for example – then this new idea can be incorporated into a subsequent nightmare, which will allow it to continue without the usual scary ending that wakes us up.

Dr Deidre Barrett believes that by using creative writing, visualization and affirmations while we are awake, we can 'incubate' the idea of a dream that we want to have while we sleep. Essentially, we can choose what we want to dream about before we go to sleep. She found that 75 per cent of participants could intentionally influence their dreams using dream incubation techniques before bed.[4]

Nightmare Rescripting combines elements from both of these approaches by inviting you to write or draw your most recent or recurrent nightmare and then to ask yourself: 'If I could change the ending of that nightmare, how would I choose it to end?'

Then in a different-coloured pen you draw (or write out) the new ending to your nightmare. Maybe you change the car crash into a new scene where the car flies away over the rooftops. Or maybe you call in one of your Circle of Protectors to protect you from a physical threat. Or maybe you summon your own inner power to transform a demon into an angel who embraces you with love.

So, in this exercise, you literally rescript and reimagine the ending however you like. Then you 'incubate' that new ending before bed through a type of hypnagogic affirmation. We'll go through it step by step below.

For some people this practice actually stops the recurring nightmares there and then, while others still have them, but now with the new ending or simply a less emotional punch.

Dr Joanne Davis explains, 'With rescription, the patient doesn't necessarily start to incorporate their new ending into their dream; instead what tends to happen is that they just don't have the nightmare, or they still have it, but it's not as powerful. Then it just decreases in frequency and goes away. It's almost as though working through the issue in the day resolves the need to relive it over and over at night.'[5]

And for some, this technique actually leads to a lucid dream in which they can consciously transform the nightmare at will.

More on lucid dreaming soon, but for now, here's a step-by-step guide to Nightmare Rescripting:

Exercise:
Nightmare Rescripting Step by Step

~ Write down or even better draw[6] your most recent or most recurrent nightmare. Allow yourself to fully download and discharge the emotional energy of the nightmare onto the page using words, images, colours and symbols. Include the feelings and emotions that you felt during the nightmare. Be creative – you can't get this wrong.

~ Take a moment to fully witness the nightmare on the page. Let the nightmare know you see it. If possible, you could even look at it and say out loud, 'I see you, nightmare.'

~ Next, ask yourself, 'If I could change the ending of that nightmare, how would I choose it to end?'

~ Then, using a different-coloured pen, write or draw however you choose to change the ending of the nightmare. Draw the car flying away from the crash, for example, or cross out the words of the usual ending and replace them with: 'I am saved by my protectors and my attacker disappears.' As always, you can't get this wrong, so be creative and don't limit yourself to realism.[7] Cognitive neuroscientist Perrine Ruby says, 'Changing the context of the dream – the laws of physics and so on – may change the perspective [and] propose another angle, a shift in our understanding which may help to change the emotion of the dream.'[8] You might even like to re-draw/re-write the newly updated dream script to further embed this new ending into your mind. For an example of this process, visit www.charliemorley.com/wakeuptosleep.

~ Then, before bed, look over the rescripted nightmare and actually rehearse it in your mind as a way of incubating it. Go through it in your head, saying, for example, 'Just before the collision the car magically flies into the sky and I am safe and free from harm.' As you do so, remind yourself that if you have that nightmare (or any other nightmare) again, you have the power to transform the ending into your chosen one.

~ Finally, as you pass through the hypnagogic, imagine the rescripted nightmare playing out, reaffirm the new ending (the car flies into the sky, for example) over and over in your mind and saturate yourself in the empowered feeling.

Daily Dosage

As and when required.

➤ Field-Tested Feedback

Keith McKenzie, the Parachute Regiment veteran to whom this book is dedicated, had such a powerful insight while doing a version of this exercise that his recurring nightmares stopped. He was actually using the technique to try and have a lucid dream, but simply the act of drawing an alternative ending to a nightmare that had plagued him for so long created some sort of resolution in his psyche that meant the nightmare never came back. He used to tease me, 'Well, I don't know if your lucid dreaming techniques work for nightmares, because I don't have them anymore!'

~ Sleep Notes ~

So many of the practices in this book can be adapted for children, and I encourage you to do so if you feel they can be of benefit. Nightmare Rescripting and Circle of Protectors are especially good, and a version of slow, deep breathing can be practised called 'Smelling the flower and blowing out the candle' in which the child inhales and exhales onto their vertically pointed index finger.

Exercise: 4-4-8 Alternate Nostril Breathing for Rapid Calming

This technique is like mental health emergency CPR and perfect for someone who has just snapped out of a night terror or sleep paralysis episode. It can even help to stop a panic attack while you are actually having one.

In this practice, you close one nostril while breathing through the other in a very specific rhythm that has been shown to induce a rapid calming effect on the mind and body.[9] A 2017 Manipal University study found that alternate nostril breathing decreased stage fright in those with a phobia of public speaking who were about to give a speech.[10] Numerous other medical studies have found that this technique rapidly lowers stress levels, heart rate and blood pressure.

These are the steps to follow:

~ Rest the second and third fingers of your right hand on the bridge of your nose, while using the thumb and pinkie finger to alternately close and release your right and left nostril in turn. If that sounds too complicated, feel free to just use one or both of your index fingers to close each nostril in turn.

~ With your right nostril closed, slowly inhale for a count of four through your left nostril. Hold your breath for count of four.

~ Now release your right nostril, close your left nostril and exhale through your right nostril for a count of eight.

~ Now Inhale through your right nostril for a count of four and hold your breath for a count of four.

~ Now release your left nostril, close your right nostril and exhale through your left nostril for a count of eight.

~ Repeat nine times or until you feel totally calm.

For a video demonstration of this technique visit www.charliemorley. com/wakeuptosleep.

Daily Dosage

As and when you need it. It can form part of a daily breathwork routine if you like.

After a few weeks of practice, you can increase the length of the exhale to a count of 10, but keep all inhalation and holding to a count of four.

~ Sleep Notes ~

I think one of the main reasons that this technique is so good for anxiety attacks is not just due to all the brain chemistry stuff, but also because it takes so much concentration to actually perform the technique that the mind is unwittingly pulled away from the anxiety overwhelm!

Exercise: Hypnopompic Mindfulness (Snooze Button Meditation)

With both night terrors and sleep paralysis most commonly happening in the hypnopompic state, learning how to stay calm and chilled within it will serve us well if and when they occur. It's also a great stand-alone mindfulness practice.

For some people, mindfulness applied in the hypnopompic can be one of the most refined experiences of pure consciousness that they have. The meditation teacher Rob Nairn is a hypnopompic specialist and it was his idea to introduce this practice into the retreats and workshops we were running together.

Rob believes, 'A level of psychological insight unmatched by any other state of mind opens up to us if we can learn how to rest in the hypnopompic.'[11]

The aim is of this practice is to become mindful of, and then rest within, that brief space between sleep and wakefulness that you pass through every time you wake up.

Here's how to do it:

~ The hypnopompic state can only be entered from full sleep, so allow yourself to wake up slowly and mindfully, without opening your eyes if possible. Don't move your body when you wake up, simply lie there mindfully aware. If it's an alarm clock that's woken you, carefully silence it or hit the snooze button, close your eyes if you opened them and re-enter the hypnopompic. (There is a buffer zone of at least a minute or so in which the hypnopompic can still be accessed after opening your eyes.)

~ Simply rest in awareness within the hypnopompic, knowing when you're breathing in and when you're breathing out. If you feel yourself slipping back into sleep, just bring yourself back to the awareness of your breath and the feeling of your body being supported by the bed.

~ Allow your mind to rest there for about five or 10 minutes (or until your snoozed alarm goes off), then open your eyes and wake up fully.

Daily Dosage

As much as you like, or every time you wake up, if possible.

~ Sleep Notes ~

You can also choose to stay in that state for hours, if you like. Rob Nairn used to practise hypnopompic mindfulness every morning from 4 a.m. to 6 a.m. and once told me that this practice gave him the core insights and ideas for his bestselling book Living, Dreaming, Dying.

Part IV Checklist ✓

✓ Remind yourself of the three new perspectives on nightmares: a dream that is shouting; the sign of a healing mind; and an evolutionary tool.

✓ Use any or all of the nightmare integration techniques as much as you like.

✓ Keep practising either Coherent Breathing or Breath–Body–Mind every day for 20 minutes minimum if you can.

✓ Keep up your regular Yoga Nidra practice too, daily if possible. If that's not possible, then as I always say: something is better than nothing.

✓ Don't scrimp on your Nocturnal Journal.

✓ Get ready to enter the mind-blowing world of lucid dreaming.

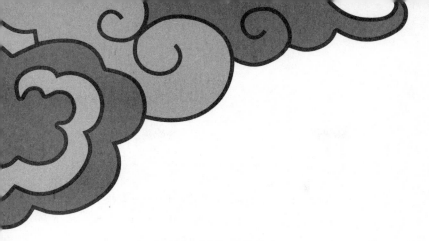

PART V

LUCID
DREAMING

'There is no greater way to profoundly shift our perception of reality than to have a lucid dream.'

ROB NAIRN, MINDFULNESS PIONEER

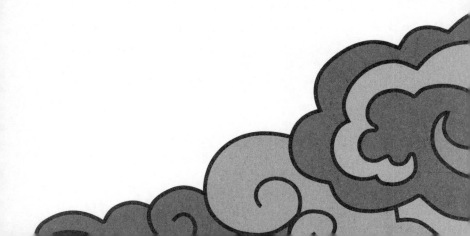

I've spent a large part of the last decade teaching people how to lucid dream and I've written two books on the subject, *Lucid Dreaming Made Easy* and *Dreams of Awakening*. I believe that lucid dreaming is without doubt one of the most powerful trauma integration treatments in existence.

But, unlike every other technique we have explored so far, it's not suitable for everyone. If you are currently working with derealization or psychosis, it will be best to wait until you have passed through the psychotic period before practising lucid dreaming.

It also might be best to wait if you are *right in the midst* of a period of trauma. This is simply because lucid dreaming takes quite a lot of effort and so you might want to stabilize your stress levels and sleep cycles before you begin.

CHAPTER 14

Making Friends with Monsters

'Once lucid, there is no need to run from what you fear. Why run from it when you can transform it?'
LAMA YESHE RINPOCHE

A lucid dream is a dream in which we know that we are dreaming as we are dreaming. Within the dream we have a sudden rush of conscious awareness in which we go, *Oh, wow, I'm dreaming! I'm in a dream right now!* and then have the ability to direct the dream at will or quite often actually wake up from the excitement. If you've ever had one of those experiences, that's a lucid dream.

From a psychological point of view, a lucid dream could be defined as 'the reactivation of self-reflective awareness within the seemingly unconscious REM dreaming sleep state', but basically it's just any dream where we know that we're dreaming as we're dreaming.

About 55 per cent of people report having had a lucid dream at least once in their lives but only 23 per cent report having them monthly,[1] so they are usually pretty rare occurrences. The good news is that lucid dreaming is a learnable skill and in Chapter 15 we'll learn everything we need to do in order to have lucid dreams.

~ Sleep Notes ~

Even if you choose not to learn the lucid dreaming practices in Chapter 15, be sure to read the Conclusion as it explains how to bring all four of the previous practices into a daily routine.

Now let's cover the basics and explore exactly how lucid dreaming can be used to transform our dreams.

Conscious within the Unconscious

In a fully lucid dream we're not half-awake, half-asleep, we're not in the hypnagogic state, and we're not having an out-of-body experience. We're sound asleep, in REM, paralysed and out for the count, but part of our brain has reactivated, allowing us to become fully conscious within our unconscious mind.

Once lucid, we become fully aware within a three-dimensional construct of our own mind. We can literally walk – or fly – around a projection of our own psychology and have complex, involved conversations with personifications of our own psyche.

Amazingly, once we are lucid, our psychological concepts are often personified, or at least animated, as dream characters. This allows us to interact with them at a seemingly physical level. We can literally have a discussion with our higher self, meet our inner child or even dialogue with the source of our deepest fear.

If being conscious within the unconscious mind sounds similar to hypnosis, it should. Essentially, anything that can be treated by hypnotherapy can also be treated by lucid dreaming: addictions, phobias, depression, confidence issues, physical ailments,[2] and of course trauma and PTSD.

And, just as a hypnotherapist might plant a beneficial suggestion of healing intent into our unconscious, so might a lucid dreamer, but due to the even deeper depths to which lucid dreaming takes us, it can work at an even deeper level.

How will you know if the lucid dream healing has worked? There will be a noticeable change in your waking-state experience – verifiable proof that it has worked.

When lucid, we can direct our dream at will and chose what we want to do, whether it's having sex with a movie star (yup, it's a thing) or healing a certain emotional wound. We can explore our unconscious mind, do spiritual practice, as in Tibetan dream yoga,[3] and even improve our sporting ability,[4] but however much we co-create the dream narrative, we never actually control the whole dream. Although we can choreograph our *subjective* dream experience, calling out for what we would like to happen or choosing to fly through the sky, the wider dreamscape is doing its own thing regardless, so we are never in full control. Nor would we want to be: lucid dreaming isn't about dominating or controlling our mind, it's about befriending it.

~ *Sleep Notes* ~

Trauma is a disempowering experience, but learning how to wake up in our dreams and direct them at will is one of the most psychologically empowering experiences there is. So, just the act of learning to lucid dream can be very helpful in counteracting the feeling of disempowered helplessness that trauma often creates.

Realer than Real

Lucid dreaming can rightly be described as 'an experience of hyper-reality'. This may seem like hyperbole, but actually it's true. The sophisticated detail of a lucid dream is mind-blowing. Put your hand on your heart when you're in one and often you'll be able to feel it beating, even though both your heart and your hand are simply the stuff that dreams are made of.

A lucid dream can even feel 'realer' than real life. This hyper-reality comes from the fact that our senses aren't limited by the constraints of our physical body. So colours may seem brighter than ever before, sounds more nuanced and touch more visceral.

THE SCIENCE OF LUCID DREAMING

Lucid dreaming has been a scientifically verified phenomenon for over 40 years. It has unique and 'discernible neural correlates', which means that it's not just psychological, it's physical.

In 2009, researchers at Frankfurt University's neurological clinic confirmed: 'Lucid dreaming constitutes a hybrid state of consciousness with definable and measurable differences from the waking state and from the REM (rapid eye movement) dream state.'[5]

Then in 2012, at Munich's Max Planck Institute of Psychiatry, using brain-monitoring equipment such as EEG and fMRI (functional magnetic resonance imaging), it was discovered that when lucid consciousness is attained within a dream, activity in 'brain areas associated with self-assessment and self-perception, including the right dorsolateral prefrontal cortex and frontopolar regions, increases markedly within seconds'.[6]

In a non-lucid dream, our sense of self, linked to activity in areas in the prefrontal cortex, is deactivated. That's why we can so easily dream we are other people or a child, for example. But what the 2012 research showed was that once we become lucidly aware and our sense of self switches back on, the prefrontal cortex becomes reactivated, proving that lucid dreaming shifts our brain into a state almost indistinguishable from waking consciousness.

The Brain Thinks You're Awake

Dreaming lucidly about doing something isn't like imagining it, it's like actually doing it. Research has found that lucid dream actions elicit the same neurological responses as actions performed while awake.[7] Holding your breath in a lucid dream, estimating time (lucid dream time and waking time feel roughly the same) and even facing fears while in a lucid dream all elicit the exact same brain responses as when awake. Studies from Heidelberg University have shown that athletes who intentionally practised their athletic discipline in their lucid dreams actually got better at it in the waking state.[8]

You know that old adage of 'Pinch yourself to see if you're dreaming'? If you pinch yourself in a lucid dream, you will simply feel pain. Even though nothing is actually being pinched (it's just your dream fingers pinching your dream arm), your brain still creates the illusion of pain. Why? Because once you're lucid, your brain thinks you're awake.

The implications of this are huge: our neurological system cannot and does not differentiate between waking and lucid dream experiences. In other words, for our brain, there is no discernible difference between lucid dream experience and waking life, so if we face a fear or integrate a trauma in a lucid dream, our brain thinks that we have actually done it in real life. That's the real USP of lucid dreaming as far as trauma integration goes.

Rewire Your Brain While You Sleep

Conscious awareness is predicated on being awake, right? Not for the brain. From a neurological point of view, self-reflective awareness is predicated on prefrontal cortex activation, regardless of what state we're in. So, to our psycho-physical system, a lucid dream isn't just a visualization, it's a reality, and because of this, neural pathways can be strengthened and created in our lucid dreams, just as they can while we are awake.

This is due to neuroplasticity: the biological basis of habit. The more we use certain brain networks, the more blood flow they receive and the deeper the grooves in the grey-matter density of that brain region become.

As we learned above, the subjective experience of lucidity – *Oh, wow, I'm dreaming!* – is accompanied by the activation of the prefrontal cortex. Once that activation occurs, our brain will start laying down new neural pathways in exactly the same way that it does when we're awake.

This means that lucid dreamers can intentionally create and strengthen neural pathways based on the actions they perform within their lucid dreams. These neural pathways will then become more easily engaged in the waking state. Lucid dreaming means that we can rewire our brain while we sleep, and so create new habits of mind, free from the debilitating affects of anxiety, stress or trauma.

Lucid Dream Trauma Integration

Over the past decade I've had the privilege of seeing how lucid dreaming can help to empower some of the most disempowered populations, from military veterans to those who were abused in childhood. But how does it actually work?

For some, it starts by working with their nightmares. About a third of all spontaneous lucid dreams begin as nightmares, and due to the awareness-boosting quality of fear, many people who have recurrent nightmares often find themselves becoming lucid within them.

The first thing most people do when they become lucid in a nightmare, though, is to try to wake themselves up. This seems logical, but it's actually missing a valuable opportunity, because when we wake ourselves up, the mental trauma or anxiety that's causing the nightmare remains unintegrated. This is why nightmares so often recur.

We need to train ourselves to stay in our nightmares, face our fears and even move towards our trauma.

How will the trauma manifest in our lucid dreams? Sometimes as a straight replay of the traumatic experience, but often the traumatized part of ourselves might take on a seemingly physicalized or personified form.

One of the unique aspects of lucid dreaming is the ability to communicate directly with these symbolic manifestations of mind. So, whether our trauma manifests as a monster rampaging towards us, a cloud of red smoke or simply a feeling of doom, rather than running from it, fighting it or rejecting it, we should remain lucid and embrace it with the compassionate realization that it is merely a mental representation of our own trauma, which we now have the valuable opportunity to integrate.

And as we learned above, if we face and integrate a trauma in a lucid dream, as far as our brain is concerned, we actually *have* integrated the trauma for real.

There are three main options available to us when using lucid dreaming to treat trauma and nightmares, but before we explore them, a note on retraumatization.

Retraumatization

Some people may be worried that intentionally facing and embracing trauma in a lucid dream may be risking retraumatization, but this is an unjustified concern. As we learned before, dreaming about painful events actually helps reduce the negative effects of difficult memories[9] and REM dreaming has been purpose-built to safely explore and integrate trauma. All we are doing through lucid dreaming is quickening that process and crucially allowing it to happen in a brain that will actually integrate the trauma just as it would if we were awake.

Also, once we're lucid, our brain simply won't allow us to do retraumatizing things: just as it will automatically pull back our hand from a fire, so it will either wake us up or simply block our request if we try to do something harmful in a lucid dream. The psychiatrist Carl Jung described this as an intelligent self-regulation mechanism in the psyche striving to maintain balance within the mind. I have seen it in action dozens of times, both in my own lucid dreams and the lucid dreams of those I've taught. Whether the mind simply ignores your request to meet the trauma or actually puts up a flashing neon sign saying 'Access denied' (that actually happened), there is no way that the evolutionary intelligence of the mind will let you go too far.

Option 1: Meeting

In this first option, we train ourselves to become lucid and then the next time we have a nightmare we intentionally try to stay in it rather than wake up.

Once lucid, we remind ourselves that our body is safe in bed and that our mind is in a place that was literally designed to explore fear and trauma: REM sleep. We are safe and ready to face our fear.

When we realize beyond doubt that what we *thought* was an external life-threatening situation is actually just a dream projection, we take the first step to integrating the nightmare.

The simple act of *intentionally* staying in the nightmare can sometimes be enough in and of itself to integrate the underlying trauma. By allowing the nightmarish manifestation of trauma to express itself and be consciously witnessed, we are allowing that energy to be witnessed, released and integrated.

Once we become lucid in a nightmare, there is also a significant shift in our brain chemistry, not only due to the reactivation of the prefrontal cortex, but also to a massive drop in stress hormone levels as we realize that we are dreaming and so not in any real danger. As we learned before, it is the elevated levels of stress hormones during REM sleep that prevents people with PTSD from gaining the healing benefits from their nightmares.

Becoming lucid significantly lowers stress hormone levels in the brain, thus allowing the healing capacity of the REM dream state to be engaged once more. Although currently unproven, I believe that this is the underlying biological mechanism of how lucid dreaming helps cure PTSD nightmares.

➤ Field-Tested Feedback

Ivan is a young man from Brazil who works as an IT researcher at the University of Copenhagen, Denmark. I met him at a lucid dreaming retreat I was running in 2018 on Holy Isle, off the west coast of Scotland. He had been having recurring nightmares, almost always about killer machines. The fear would often boost his awareness into lucidity, but he was still too scared to face them and would wake himself up if that ever happened.

Once he understood that this was what was leading to the nightmares recurring, he decided that rather than waking up he would intentionally stay in the nightmares and integrate the trauma that was creating them.

He emailed me later:

In these nightmares there are always machines that chase me and try to kill me. It's always the same theme: killer machines. In this particular nightmare there were construction site machines with mechanical arms coming to grab me. The fear made me realize it was a dream and I became fully lucid.

Once I knew I was dreaming and safe, I looked at the machines and the fear just dissolved. The nearest scary machine stopped and I imagined sending love to it, and then it slowly transformed into a tame elephant! I touched the elephant. It was a lovely animal.

Then I decided to send love to the entire dreamscape, which was a big construction site. Suddenly it all became pink, and people carrying cocktails appeared, the floor was covered with colourful flowers and the dream became like a party! I woke up smiling and I feel there has been a deep shift in my energy.

THE SCIENCE OF LUCID DREAMING FOR PTSD

There's hard science to back up all this stuff too.

A 1997 study, which took five people suffering from chronic nightmares and taught them to lucid dream, concluded that: 'The alleviation of recurrent nightmares was effective in all five cases' and 'Treatments based on lucid dream induction can be of therapeutic value.'[10]

A follow-up study a year later found that: 'Four of the five subjects no longer had nightmares and the other experienced a decrease in the intensity and frequency of their nightmares.'[11]

A 2006 study concluded that: 'Lucid dream training seems effective in reducing nightmare frequency'[12] and at the 2009 European Science Foundation meeting it was stated that lucid dreaming was such an effective remedy for nightmares that people had the potential to be 'treated by training to dream lucidly'.[13]

A 2013 neurobiological study from Brazil concluded that lucid dreaming could be used 'as a therapy for recurrent nightmares, a common symptom of post-traumatic stress disorder'.[14]

A 2019 scientific review of more than 10 different papers on lucid dream therapy (yup, it's a thing) concluded that lucid dreaming can 'aid in the treatment of patients with nightmares through minimizing their frequency, intensity and level of psychological distress'.[15]

And finally, in the summer of 2021 I was the lead facilitator of a study into PTSD treatment through lucid dreaming conducted by the Institute of Noetic Sciences in California. The study explored whether lucid dream trauma integration would be so impactful as to have an effect on inflammatory biomarkers in the body. The results will be released in 2022.

Option 2: Befriending

The second option, should it be required, is that once we become lucid, rather than just witnessing the nightmare, empowered by the knowledge that this is *our* dream and so *we* are the most powerful force within it, we proactively move towards whatever nightmarish forms or scenarios we encounter with healing intent. As I discussed in my 2011 TED talk, we literally hug them if possible, or at least psychologically face and embrace them, knowing that they are simply traumatized and wounded parts of our own psyche.[16]

And, owing to the phenomenon of neuroplasticity that occurs within lucid dreams, every time we face and embrace our fears in a lucid dream, we're strengthening the neural pathways associated with facing and embracing our fears in the waking state too.

~ Sleep Notes ~

Fascinatingly, this kind of lucid dream trauma integration also meets the requirements of what trauma expert Dr Bessel van der Kolk says is needed for trauma to be fully integrated: the reactivation of the prefrontal cortex (as we become lucid) and the regulation of the amygdala (as we face and embrace what we were afraid of).

➤ Field-Tested Feedback

A brilliant example of using recurring nightmares to become lucid and then intentionally transforming them into a dream of healing comes from my friend Ahmed.

Ahmed is an esteemed Islamic scholar who was wrongfully imprisoned over an illegal immigration claim, which led to him losing his job, his academic reputation suffering seemingly irreparable damage and a deep depression enveloping him. He experienced skin complaints and a heart problem due to the stress and soon developed emotional numbing, PTSD and recurring trauma nightmares.

He tried therapy, but it didn't help much. Then his wife bought the Arabic translation of my book *Lucid Dreaming Made Easy* for him on a hunch, thinking that lucid dreaming might help. He learned the techniques and resolved that if he became lucid within his nightmares, he would face and embrace his fears.

He emailed me from Iraq:

> *I started keeping a dream journal, did the reality checks and after a few weeks of trying, I experienced my first lucid dream.*
>
> *I was back in the country where I had been in prison and the people who had accused me were there too. At that moment I realized that I didn't live there anymore, so I had to be dreaming.*
>
> *I became lucid. I was on the main street, walking along and telling myself, 'I am dreaming — yes, I am dreaming!' I knew that within the lucid dream state I could create change that could heal me in waking life. So, in a loud and clear voice, I said, 'I am not the monster these people make me out to be. I am innocence!'*
>
> *Please note that I didn't say I was innocent, I said, 'I am innocence.' I referred directly to the quality of innocence in order to embody its truth.*
>
> *I then found myself in a park, surrounded by children playing. I felt boundless joy.*

As I was still lucid, I decided to tackle my other problem: the trauma had led me to develop an anger towards God and my practice of prayer had become very irregular. So I took the opportunity to mend my relationship with God. With the innocence of a child, I called out to the dream: 'I love God so much! I am just too hurt.'

I was flooded by boundless limitless love and moved to tears of joy, and red flowers started growing all around me. And then I woke up.

It has been three months since that lucid dream. The eczema is gone, the fits of rage are gone, the ruminating about the past is gone. My wife tells me that the difference in me is that of night and day.

I am at peace now. I know I have done nothing wrong and I am more optimistic about the future, more creative.

In that one single dream I was able to heal the two big wounds that had poisoned my life. I am no longer angry at God. I know I am loved and that these trials all had a wisdom.

Ahmed's lucid dream healing is a profound example of the power of lucid dream treatment for PTSD and trauma. When I read his words, I feel even more confident that one day in my lifetime, lucid dream therapy will be offered as widely and respected as highly as any other form of psychotherapy.

•••

Option 3: Transforming

In option number three, we don't wait for the nightmare to happen, we intentionally seek out its source and call it to us.

Once lucid, we call the source of our trauma or wounding into the dream in order to bear witness to it, embrace it with love and perhaps even dialogue with it too.

In the dream, we literally call out, for example: 'I want to meet my sexual shame!' or 'I am ready to release my childhood trauma. Childhood trauma, I release you!' And then, whatever appears, whether a personification of the trauma, a monster of misplaced shame, or simply a feeling of doom, we embrace it with loving acceptance, either literally or with our intent.

If we can do that, then we can, as a Jungian psychotherapist attending one of my retreats once told me, 'heal more trauma in one lucid dream than in years of therapy'.

So, although it might take weeks or even months to get to the point where our lucid dream training is stable enough for us to turn to face a trauma in a lucid dream, once we do that, we might wake up the next morning feeling like a very different person.

➤ Field-Tested Feedback

Fiona had been a psychiatric nurse for over 30 years when I first met her. She came to various courses that I was running, including lucid dreaming ones, and a Shadow integration one too. She had started having nightmares a few years earlier, due to the resurfacing of childhood trauma combined with PTSD from being knocked down by a car 20 years before. She was also having regular false awakenings with sleep paralysis and night terrors, but she soon started having amazing success with the various techniques she learned. In her words:

The first time I managed to transform trauma was during a recurring nightmare about a male figure entering my room. I became lucid and managed to confront him, and I actually said, 'I love you,' to him. I knew that this was what he needed to hear, because he was just a part of me that was wounded.

Once I said those words, he disappeared in a burst of black smoke that was sucked up and out of the dream.

I thought that might be the end of it, but there are layers to trauma, I suppose, because I had another nightmare a week or so later, and this time saying 'I love you' didn't work and I woke up with my husband comforting me.

Nothing happened for about five weeks, but I was so anxious every night that I had to use Yoga Nidra and my Circle of Protectors just to get to sleep.

After our last chat, though, I felt ready to face whatever it was that the figure represented.

That night, when I'd visualized my protection circle around me, in my head I actually invited the nightmare figure to come into my dreams that night. And he did come and I did become lucid, but this time I was ready.

When I became lucid, he was standing over me and I just said, 'I've been waiting for you. Can we be friends?'

Suddenly the dark figure turned white and dissolved in front of me like icing sugar falling to the floor.

The next day I woke feeling really tired, and also hungover, though I'd had no alcohol. Then a kind of euphoria hit me and I realized just what I'd managed to do.

Since then I haven't been terrified to go to sleep and if the nightmares do return, then I know what to do!

Fiona's story offers a textbook example not only of using all the different tools in the toolbox of techniques, but also of how we can harness our inner courage to face and embrace our nightmares. The hungover feeling she described was significant too: she had obviously released something at a deep somatic level.

•••

We can work with seemingly more everyday (but often just as debilitating) wounds through lucid dreaming too. Because this is a book about stress- and trauma-affected sleep, the examples that I am choosing are mostly reflective of that theme, but the vast majority of lucid dreamers become lucid not through nightmares, but simply through learning how to have lucid dreams. Once they know how to lucid dream, they can then use their lucidity to work with creative blocks, relationship issues, sports training and even diet issues.

➤ Field-Tested Feedback

Robert came to one of the online lucid dreaming retreats that I ran during the 2020 lockdowns and wanted to work with his unhealthy relationship to food. We had discussed how the psychological term 'the Shadow' referred to anything within us that we had repressed, denied or disowned – often shame, fears and trauma. So, Robert wanted to integrate the Shadow of his unhealthy relationship to food.

He made a dream plan (a technique that we will learn in the next chapter for planning out a lucid dream you intend to have), practised the lucid dreaming techniques as he fell asleep, and once he was lucid, this is what happened:

I called out, 'Eating Shadow, come to me!'

Then to my right I noticed a young man lying on the ground next to me. I looked at his head and I could see a large tongue curling around out of a slit in the side of his forehead.

I asked, 'Are you my Eating Shadow?' and he said, 'Yes.'

I went to embrace him, but I could see other people looking at us intently. I asked him, 'Are these people my Shadow as well?' and he said, 'Yes,' so I called out to everyone, 'Let's have a group hug!' and they all came forward and surrounded me.

I stretched my arms out to embrace everyone and I could barely fit my arms around them all. It was amazing. I was actually hugging my Eating Shadow.

I woke up with a feeling that this was the most incredible experience of my life. And it did change my life too.

The next day, my wife, Anne, and I were out for a meal and she noticed with surprise that I had left half of my main course uneaten. She asked if it was okay.

I said it was lovely, but I didn't need to eat any more of it. That had never happened before.

I still like my food, but I'm now selective about my portion size and I no longer feel controlled by the urge to overeat or go to the cupboard for something to eat as a way of suppressing my emotions. It's been a big change for me and a profound healing too.

•••

Lucid Dreaming Therapy

Lucid dreaming has massive potential as a therapeutic tool and I believe that there will come a time when we will have full-time lucid dream therapists whose job will be to advise patients on how they can work with own psyche directly through their lucid dreams.

I want to give the final word on this possibility to James Scurry, a rare combination of qualified psychotherapist and person who has used lucid dreaming as a therapeutic tool himself. At a workshop that I was giving, he spoke to participants about his personal experiences with lucid dreaming and how he thought it could fit into the mainstream psychotherapeutic model:

I wanted to combine my psychotherapist training with lucid dreaming because I think that we're only just beginning to understand how powerful lucid dreaming is and I wanted to explore it for myself.

I had been trying to work with my own childhood trauma in the therapy sessions I was having, but I couldn't access it in the therapy room. It was just endless talking and I found that I would get triggered and it just wasn't working.

So I made a dream plan to meet my inner child. I learned the techniques, and when I next became lucid, I called out to meet my inner child with the intention of healing the childhood trauma.

He appeared sitting on the bed — just this little boy with blond hair. He had been locked in that room, though, all alone, and he was sick.

There wasn't any fanfare to it, it wasn't like some kind of big epiphany. He didn't even talk, actually. But the thing was, I got to hold him, to hug him. I got to feel how small he was.

And my heart just completely cracked open. And I just talked to him. I told him that I was so sorry. And then I just woke up with tears streaming down my face. It was an incredible healing.

It was then that I began to understand the true implications of this practice. I am a psychotherapist myself, but I couldn't contact that wounded little boy through my therapy sessions, I could only do it through the lucid dream state. In one night of lucid dreaming, I did what I wouldn't have been able to do in hundreds of hours of therapy.

So, if lucid dreaming really does offer us such profound benefits, let's waste no time in learning how to do it...

CHAPTER 15

Lucid Dreaming Practices

'There are three essential requirements for learning lucid dreaming: adequate motivation, correct practice of effective techniques, and excellent dream recall.'

DR STEPHEN LABERGE, EXPERT IN THE SCIENTIFIC
STUDY OF LUCID DREAMING

The following techniques have been abridged from my second book, *Lucid Dreaming Made Easy*, but I have added to them and adapted them for a readership working with stress or trauma.

Lucid dreaming can take weeks or months to stabilize, and even then we may only be having a few fully lucid dreams a month, but we only need one lucid dream to change our life, so the effort is definitely worth it.

This is quite a big practice, so I'll explain all the techniques first and then how to put them together in a week-by-week practice.

Take it slowly, be sure to keep up the other core practices – sleep awareness, rest and relaxation, breathwork and nightmare integration – and enjoy learning how to lucid dream.

Exercise: Lucid Dream Planning

The first thing you need to do is to focus on the 'why'. Why do you want to have a lucid dream? Having a good reason to have a lucid dream is the most powerful lucid dreaming technique there is.

When you set a strong intention to do something in your next lucid dream, you not only start to attract the causes and conditions needed to make that dream manifest, but also create the expectation of becoming lucid.

On my workshops I teach lucid dream planning in three main stages: i) writing a dream plan; ii) drawing a dream plan (the dreaming mind works in images, so this helps); and iii) creating a *sankalpa* (a Sanskrit term meaning 'will or purpose'), or statement of intent. The steps below include them all.

~ Draft some ideas of what you'd like to do in your next lucid dream. What would you like to heal? What trauma would you like to integrate? What part of your Shadow would you like to interact with?

~ Once you've decided what you want to do, begin to formulate your dream plan. Start with 'In my next lucid dream I...' and then write a description of what you want to do once lucid.

~ Next, draw a picture of your dream plan in action. I just use stick men and speech bubbles, but if you're artistic, then of course feel free to do more.

~ Now write your *sankalpa*, or statement of intent. This should be a pithy statement that sums up the essence of your dream plan. For example, if my dream plan is a complex description of how I want to meet my relationship anxiety and embrace it with loving-kindness, my *sankalpa* might be much more concise: 'Heartbroken Charlie, come to me!' Your dream plan can be as long and detailed as you like, but I recommend that you keep your *sankalpa* short and sharp.

~ The final step occurs when you next find yourself in a lucid dream. Once you get lucid, recall your dream plan, say your *sankalpa* out loud and then carry out your chosen dream plan.

In my next lucid dream I will...
Heal the wounded part of myself by calling out within the dream:
'I am healed! I am free of my wounds! Wounded self, I release you!'
As this happens, I experience a deeply beneficial integration of my
psychological wounds and wake up feeling peaceful and healed.

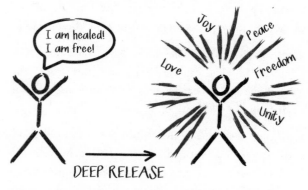

DEEP RELEASE

Sankalpa: 'I am healed! I am free of my wounds!'
'Wounded self, I release you!'

My dream plan

Sometimes the dream planning technique can plant such strong seeds of intent that our unconscious mind responds to our request and we become lucid, but usually we need to create a few more conditions to help foster lucid dreams.

Here are a few of the most effective ways to do so...

Exercise: Dream Recall and Documenting Your Dreams

I hope you are still keeping your Nocturnal Journal. Writing down your sleep experience each night helps to solidify the memory of a mainly unconscious process into your conscious awareness. Each time you do this, you are not only strengthening those sleep awareness muscles (making each journal entry easier to make), but you are also strengthening that line of communication between your unconscious and conscious mind. The stronger that line of communication becomes, the stronger your mental health may become too.

Training yourself to be able to recall and remember your dreams is essential to lucid dreaming because the more conscious you are *of* your dreams, the easier it will be to become conscious *within* your dreams.

Most people have four or five dream periods every night, but not everybody remembers them. I believe the main reason is simply because we don't *try* to remember them. So, the first thing you need to do is to set a strong intention to remember your dreams. If you do this, you should be able to recall at least part of them without too much difficulty after just a couple of nights. After all, four or five dream periods a night means about 1,800 dreams periods per year and well over 100,000 dreams periods in a lifetime! Oh, and each dream period might contain multiple dreams. So you'll have plenty of dreams to remember...

The next step is to document them when you wake up from them, either in your Nocturnal Journal or in a newly purposed dream diary.

~ Before bed, and again as you're falling asleep (through the hypnotically suggestible hypnagogic state), recite over and over in your mind for at least a couple of minutes: *Tonight, I remember my dreams. I have excellent dream recall.* This simple method can be a profoundly effective remedy for dream amnesia.

~ Whenever you wake up from a dream, recall as much of it as you can and then write it down or document it in some way. You don't need to record every tiny detail – you'll know what feels worth noting and what doesn't – and you don't need to spend ages on this either. Just focus on the main themes and feelings and the general narrative. If you can recall just one fact or feeling from your dream, you can work backwards from that point and eventually gather the rest of the dream.

~ Often our memories of our dreams are felt in our body rather than logged solely in our mind, so don't forget to explore any feelings in your body that you wake up with. Sometimes my dream recollection is as simple as: 'Can't remember much of the dream, but I woke with a feeling of happiness in my belly.'

Daily Dosage

If possible, recite the dream recall affirmation every time you fall asleep and write in your dream diary every morning.

Unless you are writing down your dreams at least four or five times a week, it may be a long road to lucidity.

Top Tips for Documenting Your Dreams

- Write: 'Woke up with no dream recall' if you can't remember any dreams, as this will at least help foster the habit of keeping a dream diary every morning.

- Don't give up on recalling a dream if you can't remember it straight away. Give yourself space to remember.

- If you choose to use your smartphone as your dream diary, be sure to turn down the screen brightness.

- I rarely spend more than five or 10 minutes writing down my dreams when I wake, but I often expand them over breakfast. You might like to do the same.

Once you start regularly recalling and documenting your dreams, you may start to see repeating elements emerging. You might notice that you often dream of your dead grandma or of being back in your childhood home, for example, or that you dream of being chased by zombies at least once a week.

These repeating elements can be used to become lucid, because once you become aware of them in the waking state, you might also become aware of them while dreaming and go, *Hang on, I always dream of zombies. Wait – oh wow, I must be dreaming right now!*

This forms the basis of our next technique: dream signs.

Exercise: Dream Signs

A dream sign is any improbable, impossible or bizarre aspect of dream experience that can indicate we're dreaming. Most people's dreams are full of dream signs – things as far out as talking dogs and dead relatives or as subtle as being back at school. Basically, if it's something that doesn't usually occur in waking life, it may well be a dream sign.

I classify dream signs into three main groups:

~ Anomalous: random, one-off anomalies such as talking fish or ninja babies.

~ Thematic: dreamlike themes or scenarios such as being back at school or being naked in public.

~ Recurring: dream signs that have appeared multiple times. These are a real boon for lucid dreamers.

One of the most important reasons for keeping a dream diary is to record and chart our personal dream signs. Once we know what they are, the next time we see one in a dream, it can trigger lucidity.

Spotting Dream Signs

~ Once you've recalled and written down your dreams, read back through them, on the lookout for dream signs. If you dreamed that you were walking down a street and saw Barack Obama standing next to a blue dragon, for example, then your dream signs would be 'Barack Obama' and 'blue dragon'. Unless you were Michelle Obama, of course, in which case seeing Barack Obama wouldn't be a dream sign, because he would be a feature of your everyday life. The blue dragon, however, would still be a dream sign. If you'd dreamed of a blue dragon several times, it would be a recurring dream sign. Recurring dream signs mean recurring opportunities to become lucid!

~ Once you've pinpointed your dream signs, set a strong intention to recognize them the next time they show up. Before bed, remind yourself again and again: 'The next time I see a blue dragon, I'll know that I'm dreaming!' Then, when you next dream about your dream sign, the lucidity trigger will be activated, making you spontaneously think, *Blue dragon? Aha! This is a dream sign — I must be dreaming!* And you'll become lucid.

Once you start noticing your dream signs, you may find that you start having dreams full of them. This is a good sign, because it shows that your unconscious mind is trying to help you become lucid by sending loads of crazy dream signs into your dreams!

Daily Dosage

Every time you write down a dream, check through it to spot your dream signs. Eventually this process will become automatic, but in the early stages you might like to make a list of your current dream signs.

~ Sleep Notes ~

Every time we recognize and acknowledge a dream sign as we read through our dreams, we create and strengthen a habit of critical reflective awareness, which soon seeps into our dreams. That is what gets us lucid!

Spotting a dream sign is one of the most common ways into a lucid dream. But sometimes, even though we've spotted a dream sign and are sure that we must be dreaming, the rest of the dream looks so realistic that we simply can't accept that we're in a dream.

This is when we need a reality check.

Exercise: Reality Checks

Dr Stephen LaBerge and the researchers at the Lucidity Institute in California have scientifically verified that there are certain things that are virtually impossible for the human mind to replicate consistently in the pre-lucid dream state (the state just before we're lucid),[1] and so these can be used to confirm whether or not we're dreaming.

Reality checks are performed within the non-lucid dream state, but of course if we're conscious enough to think, *I should do a reality check*, then we're almost lucid already.

There are lots of different reality checks, but I'll take you through some of my favourites. Can you do the following? If not, then you might be dreaming:

~ Look at your outstretched hand twice in quick succession without it changing in some way.

~ Read text coherently twice without it changing in some way.

~ Use digital or electrical devices without them changing or malfunctioning in some way.

During a dream, our brain is working flat out to maintain our elaborately detailed dreamscape in real time, and although it's amazingly good at this, once we're pre-lucid, it often struggles to replicate the detail of an intricate image, such as a piece of text or an outstretched hand, twice in quick succession. So, if we try to make it engage in such a replication, it will provide a close but imperfect rendering, and it's the acknowledgement of this imperfect rendering that makes us lucid.

Let's explore those three reality checks in more depth:

Looking at Your Hands

If something weird has just happened and you think you might be dreaming, but you're not 100 per cent sure, look at your outstretched hand, then quickly look away and look back at it again. Alternatively, watch your hand as you flip it over and back again.

Either way, your dreaming mind will try its best to reproduce exactly the same image, but it doesn't quite have the processing speed to do so perfectly, so on second glance your hand may be a strange shape, perhaps missing a finger or two, or look dappled or transformed. I've seen my hand turn into a baby elephant and grow three new fingers!

Reading Text

In a dream, it's virtually impossible to read any text coherently twice in succession. LaBerge's research laboratory found that even in lucid dreams, text changed 75 per cent of the time as the dreamer was reading it and 95 per cent of the time on second reading.[2] So, if you think you might be dreaming, try to read something. The text will often be unintelligible, move around as you're reading it, or in some cases just fade away altogether. All these are signs that you're dreaming.

Using Digital or Electrical Appliances

Just as the dreaming mind struggles to reproduce text, it also struggles with the highly detailed screen of a smartphone or a computer, which will often seem blurred and transformed in some way. I know it sounds crazy, but in a dream it's often impossible to read a digital watch, successfully operate any form of digital or electrical appliance or even switch a light on and off.

Although opportunities for reality checks will often crop up in your dreams, you'll usually only take them when you've spotted a dream sign and need confirmation of your present reality.

You can, however, actively hasten the process by getting into the habit of conducting reality checks while you're awake. That's the basis of the Weird Technique.

~ Sleep Notes ~

If you think you might be dreaming but want to be 100 per cent sure (before you try to fly through the sky), look at anything with a detailed pattern, such as your hand, twice in a row, and if it changes, you'll know for sure that you're dreaming.

Exercise: The Weird Technique

This is a deceptively simple technique through which I have the majority of my lucid dreams. Here's how to do it:

~ As you go about your daily life, whenever something weird happens, or whenever you experience synchronicity, *déjà vu*, a strange coincidence or any other type of dreamlike anomaly, take a moment to think, *That's weird. Could I be dreaming right now?*

~ Then perform a reality check, and as long as your hand doesn't grow an extra finger or morph into a baby elephant, you can be sure that you're not dreaming.

This sets up a habit that'll crop up in your dreams too, but in your dreams your hand *will* change and you'll become lucid.

Daily Dosage

Practise it every day if you can. Every time you see something weird or unexpected, notice it and do a reality check.

Until you start doing 10 or more Weird Technique reality checks per day, the habit may not start to enter into your dreams.

All of the lucid dreaming techniques so far have been what in the Tibetan Buddhist tradition we would call 'daytime techniques', because we do them in the daytime while we are awake. The next two techniques are classed as 'night-time techniques', because we do them as we are falling asleep at night.

Exercise: Hypnagogic Affirmation

In this technique, as you fall asleep through the hypnagogic state, you harness the hypnotic potential of this state by mentally reciting a positive affirmation of your intent to gain lucidity.

You can do this as you first fall asleep, but for best results practise it after an early-hours wake-up – at least four-and-a-half to five hours after you went to bed – so that you don't interrupt your deep sleep periods. The last few hours of our sleep cycle are also when we enter dreams most easily from the waking state and at this time the hypnagogic will lead directly into the dream state.

If you are currently experiencing high levels of stress, anxiety or heartache, you may find that if you wake up, you may not be able to get back to sleep. If that keeps happening, then only practise this technique as you first fall asleep.

Whenever you practise it, though, the important thing is to saturate your sleepy consciousness with your intention to have a lucid dream.

~   Take some time to create an affirmation such as: 'I recognize my dreams with full lucidity,' or 'Next time I'm dreaming, I know that I'm dreaming,' or whatever phrase you feel best encapsulates your intention to get lucid.

~   As you enter the hypnagogic state, continuously recite this affirmation in your mind. Try to do it with real feeling and gusto – this is vital, because without determination, this technique simply won't work.

~   Keep reciting. The important thing is not so much that you're repeating the affirmation right up to the point at which you enter a dream (although that would be great), but more that you saturate your last few minutes of conscious awareness with the strong intention to gain lucidity. Aim for your affirmation to be the last thing to pass through your mind before you black out.

Daily Dosage

Every night if you like, but be careful that the technique doesn't disrupt your sleep too much. The affirmation should only be recited for a few minutes as you are falling asleep and no longer than that.

If you wake up to pee at nights, that gives you a perfect and non-disruptive chance to practise this technique as you fall back asleep.

Exercise: Falling Asleep Consciously (FAC)

For many people, falling asleep consciously is the Holy Grail of lucid dreaming practice, but it's really not such a big deal. Although it can take a long time to master it, I've taught it to hundreds of people and seen them apply it successfully within a few weeks, or even on the first night of practice.

The aim is to pass through the hypnagogic state and enter REM dreaming sleep without blacking out or losing consciousness. This is both incredibly simple and often incredibly elusive, and involves letting your body and brain fall asleep while part of your mind stays aware.

This technique combines elements of a well-known lucid dreaming technique called WILD (wake-initiated lucid dream) with a few of my own methods and a twist of meditative awareness. Again, it is best practised after briefly waking in the last few hours of your sleep cycle. If you wake in the early hours, either naturally or with an alarm, and then fall back asleep, you'll enter the dream state much more quickly than earlier in the night, and for this technique it's a case of the more direct the entry into the dream state, the better.

But again, if you find that stress or a racing mind prevents you from falling asleep, then stop practising this technique.

I have two favourite versions of the FAC technique. Let's look at each one individually.

Hypnagogic Drop-in

Here you're like a surfer: you paddle through the hypnagogic imagery and lucidly 'drop in' to the wave of the dream. If you've a good sense of mental balance and awareness, then this is the technique for you!

~   After at least four-and-a-half to five hours of sleep, wake up and write down your dreams. Then set your intent to gain lucidity, close your eyes and allow yourself to drift back to sleep.

~   As you enter the hypnagogic state, gently focus on the imagery and simply float through it, allowing it to build, layer upon layer, until it starts to coalesce into an actual dreamscape. The key here is to maintain a delicate vigilance without blacking out and being sucked into the dream state unconsciously.

~   As the dreamscape solidifies, you might feel a slight pull or a sensation of being sucked forwards. This is an indication that the wave of the dream is now fully formed. In surfing terms, you're on point break.

~   If you can just stay conscious for a few more moments and are ready to take the plunge, you'll find yourself dropping into the wave of the dream with full lucidity.

Body and Breath

If you have good body awareness (perhaps you like to dance, or do body work or yoga), you may find that this version of the FAC technique is the one for you.

~ Sometime after at least four-and-a-half to five hours of sleep, wake up and write down your dreams. Set your intent to gain lucidity, close your eyes and allow yourself to drift back to sleep.

~ As you enter the hypnagogic state, gently focus on the sensations in your body and the breath flowing through it. Hypnagogic imagery will arise, but continue to focus on the sensations in your body. If you feel yourself blacking out, just keep bringing your focus back to the sensations of your body and breath. You might find that systematically scanning through your body works well for this. Alternatively, you might choose simply to allow bodily sensations to attract your attention as they arise. Becoming aware of the contact points of your body on the bed works well too.

~ At some point you may actually feel the body paralysis that accompanies REM sleep. There's no need to freak out if this happens – it simply means that you're at the doorway of a dream.

~ Become aware of your whole body as it lies in space and remain aware as the dream forms out of the hypnagogic. Then you'll enter it lucidly.

Daily Dosage

As much as you like, as long as it doesn't disrupt your sleep too much.

Creating a Practice

Put all those techniques together and you have a fully-fledged lucid dreaming practice! Here's exactly how to do it.

Once you've made your dream plan, you might want to spend at least the next week just concentrating on your dream recall and documenting your dreams, so that you have a really firm basis for your practice. Aim to be recalling at least one dream a night if you can.

Solid dream recall also means solid dream sign recognition, because the more dreams you recall, the more dream signs you'll notice.

Once you start to become aware of your dream signs, you might start to become aware of them *while you are dreaming*, which may well lead to your first lucid dream. Spend the next week or so really focusing on recognizing your dream signs.

This is where reality checks come in, as sometimes even though we recognize a dream sign, the rest of the dream looks so realistic that we just can't believe that we're actually dreaming. That's exactly the situation in which to perform a reality check.

How will you actually remember to do reality checks in your dreams? By getting into the habit of doing them while you're awake: the Weird Technique. You can either start doing this straight away or after a week or two of focusing mainly on dream recall and dream signs.

Add to all this the two night-time practices, hypnagogic affirmation and falling asleep consciously, and you'll have a pretty solid lucid dreaming practice.

Some of you will get lucid tonight simply from the enthused determination to do so, whereas others will take a couple of weeks to have their first lucid dream.

At an in-person weekend workshop I will teach all the lucid dreaming techniques above in just two days, whereas on an online course I will spread them out over six weeks, so feel free to set your own schedule and take it at your own pace.

If you want to go deeper into lucid dreaming and learn dozens of other induction techniques, you might like to check out all my courses and workshops at www.charliemorley.com.

Lucid Living

Before we conclude our chapters on lucid dreaming, I want to plant the seed of another brilliant side-effect of lucidity: lucid living.

The Tibetan Buddhist master Traleg Rinpoche once said, 'Through lucid dreaming we plant seeds which will manifest in the conscious mind. If we can learn to transform our nightmares, we will not only wake up with more resilience, but we will be able to transform the nightmares of our daily lives too.'[3]

We live as we dream, and so every time we face, embrace and integrate a trauma in a lucid dream, we create a habitual tendency to do the same while awake. Every time we fly through the sky in a lucid dream, we are creating a new mental habit of moving beyond limitation in our waking life. Every time we face a fear in a lucid dream, we are creating a new mindset in our waking life that says, 'I am no longer limited by fear.' Lucid dreaming thus leads to lucid living – to transformation of both our night and our day.

Part V Checklist ✓

✓ Writing down your dreams (every morning if possible or at least five days out of seven) and doing reality checks during the day are essential if you want to have lucid dreams.

✓ Make sure that your dream plan makes you salivate. It should excite you and make you want to go to bed early. If your dream plan isn't pretty life-changing, then create a one that is. Go deep!

✓ If your sleep has stabilized enough to do the brief wake-ups required for the hypnagogic affirmation technique and falling asleep consciously – and, crucially, if anxiety isn't preventing you from falling back asleep – then be sure to use these techniques a few times a week at least.

✓ Regardless of whether you are doing the lucid dreaming techniques or not, keep practising either Coherent Breathing or Breath-Body-Mind every day for at least 20 minutes, plus your regular Yoga Nidra practice.

✓ Use the nightmare integration techniques as you like and feel free to use the breathing exercises (the 4,7,8 Breath and Alternate Nostril Breathing), regardless of whether or not you are having nightmares.

✓ Check out the next chapter for advice on how to integrate all of the practices in this book into your everyday life.

Conclusion

'A year ago today I was on the veterans' retreat.
Since then I've gone from five nightmares a week
to zero. Only woken up with the terrors once in
the past year. Thanks, Charlie and Keith!'
FACEBOOK POST FROM BRIAN, A SCOTTISH VETERAN

As the roaring 20s of this new millennium offer unprecedented new challenges, as well as brave new opportunities, one thing is for sure: our ability to cope with them will be written in the lines under our eyes.

Will we thrive or merely survive? Sleep will play a large part in the answer to that question. The first and most obvious manifestation of stress and trauma is disturbed sleep. While awake, we might be convinced that we're coping with stress or unaware of how an unintegrated trauma is draining us, but once the light goes out, all is revealed.

And, as we learned before, when working with stress or trauma, we need stronger medicine than sleep hygiene hacks. We need to treat the root cause: a dysregulated nervous system.

As we learned in the first chapter, every one of our biological processes is negatively affected by poor sleep, but enhanced by sleeping well. And sleeping well is our birthright.

Creating a Practice in Everyday Life

Although originally developed for British military veterans, the practices in this book have been adapted to be suitable for anyone with stressed-out sleep. They are tried and tested techniques. Both Breath-Body-Mind and Yoga Nidra have been used to successfully treat PTSD in some of the most traumatized populations for decades now. And lucid dreaming is such a promising new treatment for trauma that there have been more scientific studies conducted on this subject in the past 10 years than in the previous 50. At the time of writing, I'm about to begin lead facilitation in a new study at the Institute of Noetic Sciences, founded by the brilliant Dr Dean Radin, looking at the effectiveness of lucid dreaming for PTSD trauma integration. This is happening as we await the publication of a successful 2019 Swansea University study on the same topic. Lucid dreaming really is at the cutting edge of trauma research.

Once you start practising breathwork, hypnagogic mindfulness and lucid dreaming, while adding nightmare integration techniques and sleep awareness into the mix, you end up with a very effective protocol.

And although many of you will already have felt the benefits of one or all of these practices, it can take a while for both our body and mind to adjust to them, so give them time. Remember, this book is based upon the Mindfulness of Dream & Sleep six-week course, so give yourself at least six to eight weeks for the practices to take root.

In fact, you might even like to spend a whole week or more focusing on one of the five foundational practices before moving on to the next: a whole week of just keeping your Nocturnal Journal before taking a whole week to really get to grips with Yoga Nidra practices, then spending a solid seven days on Coherent Breathing and so on.

You don't have to do all of the techniques all the time, though. This book should be seen as a toolbox of techniques. Choose your favourite tools and feel free to create a personal practice that works for you.

Here are a few practice routines based on the different character types that I've encountered at my workshops:

- The Bed Lover: a few minutes of Nocturnal Journaling in the morning to start the day, a 15-minute powernap underneath the desk at lunch and 30 minutes of Yoga Nidra every evening after work.

- The Breath Enthusiast: Thirty minutes of coherent breathing or Breath-Body-Mind every day, alternate nostril breathing before a big Zoom meeting at work and the 4-7-8 breath to chill out before bed. Plus mouth-taping while asleep to encourage nasal breathing.

- The Lucid Dreamer: Dream diary every morning, reality checks during the day, 4 a.m. wake-ups twice a week to practise the lucid dreaming techniques and a wide-eyed enthusiasm for lucid dreaming.

- The Nightmare Experiencer: Nocturnal Journaling every morning, 20 minutes of Coherent Breathing before bed, 10 minutes of deep relaxation while in bed and the Circle of Protectors while falling asleep. The 4-7-8 breath or alternate nostril breathing if waking after an upsetting dream, plus awareness of lucid dream techniques in case of lucidity in a nightmare.

But what about those working with trauma or PTSD? The ideal programme could be:

- 2 × 20-minute sessions of Breath-Body-Mind/Coherent Breathing every day

- at least 20 minutes of Yoga Nidra every day

- at least 10 minutes of deep relaxation before bed (or any of the techniques from Chapter 5)

- daily Nocturnal Journaling

- use of nightmare integration techniques when applicable

- after six to eight weeks (or whenever sleep has stabilized), gradual introduction of lucid dreaming practices

For some who are working with trauma, that might seem a totally unrealistic programme, and for many it will be, so see it simply as an ideal to aspire to rather than an obligation to worry about. Trauma often dials down both our motivation and our energy levels, so be kind to yourself. If just five minutes of slow, deep breathing is all you do some days, then that's totally okay. Other days, when your motivation is up, you might do a full 20-minute Coherent Breathing session and some Yoga Nidra too. Both days can be celebrated.

Just managing to get out of bed in the morning can be celebrated if you're working with depression or trauma. There are no rules to this thing – use the tools in your toolbox as you see fit, but if you can aspire to do at least 20 minutes of something, be that breathwork or Yoga Nidra, each day, that would be great.

The most important tip for everyone is to use what works for you. For some people, just 20 minutes of Coherent Breathing a day will change their life; for others, it may be the revelation that lying down on the floor in a semi-sleep state for half an hour a day isn't only the most wonderfully relaxing practice, but also completely chills them out and has a massively positive effect on their sleep cycle. For others, it may be the lucid dreaming practices that they really connect with, as they realize that if they can integrate the root cause of their trauma in a lucid dream, then that in itself will regulate their waking-state nervous system and allow them to sleep better.

It's all about 'horses for courses', so make your practice your own and feel free to use whatever combination you feel is best. Each one of the five core practices is a powerful way to treat stress and trauma-affected sleep in and of itself, so whether you choose to practise all of them every day, a few of them each week, or to put all your focus on the one that you really resonate with, the results will speak for themselves, so you'll soon see what works best for you.

I received an email from a young woman called Emma, who attended the six-week course that this book is based on, which really sums this up. She said:

> *I'm feeling so positive now. Not just because I have a bunch of new tools in my tool box, but because I no longer feel like a freak and I am no longer scared about having nightmares. I don't feel broken anymore and I have actually felt confident enough to talk about exploring my past trauma.*
>
> *It feels like I'm finally getting to the root cause and not just tackling the symptoms. I can't tell you how happy that makes me feel.*
>
> *I know I still have work to do and it might take time but I feel like I have the final piece of my puzzle: the course, the five practices, how they all work together... they have had such a big impact.*

If you start experiencing better sleep quality, less daytime stress and anxiety, increased energy levels, a change in your perception of nightmares and, crucially, a friendlier relationship with sleep, then keep doing whatever you're doing. If not, then feel free to tweak the combination of practices to find what works for you.

And finally, you can always expand your practice with me in person or online. Come and join a live workshop or retreat, take an online course or check out the free Lucid Dream Drop-Ins that I run each month. The details for all of these can be found at www.charliemorley.com. Scholarships are always available for veterans and those who are struggling financially.

The Way Ahead

The last 10 years have seen mindfulness move from the fringe to the mainstream, with it now being offered by schools, national health systems, military training programmes and international governments.

Over the same period, a growing interest in sleep science has become mainstream too, with terms like 'sleep hygiene' and 'sleep hacking' cropping up in water-cooler conversations comparing 'sleep-tracker' data from the night before.

And yet these two zeitgeists haven't yet been fully integrated. My hope is that this book has helped in some way to do that.

There are of course dozens of books exploring each of the five core practices that make up the Mindfulness of Dream & Sleep programme, but this is, to my knowledge, the first to bring all of them together into one book with a trauma-sensitive approach.

Dr Daniel Libby is a clinical psychologist and the founder of the Veterans' Yoga Project in the Bay Area of California. As part of my Winston Churchill Fellowship research I interviewed him about his work, and he told me, 'Trauma, at its core, is a disempowering experience. Post-Traumatic Stress is a disempowering disorder. The practices of breathing and working with your body are about re-empowering you. They're about connecting you with your own mind, your own body, your own will and your ability to live and to value your life.'[1]

I truly hope that the practices in this book help you to do just that and that you can use them to re-empower your relationship to those 30 years that you spend asleep in order to be, as my Buddhist teacher Lama Yeshe Rinpoche once said: 'More awake, more aware. More aware, more kind. More kind to yourself and others: that's the point!'

Sleep Hygiene Practices

As we learned earlier, most of the sleep hygiene and sleep hacking approaches to sleeplessness are based around changing the external conditions (the weather) of sleep, rather than the root cause (the climate). That being said, though, let's cover a few of the most effective sleep hygiene tips, just so we can have them in our toolbox.

One of the main reasons that I don't place much emphasis on sleep hygiene hacks in general is that they often create an additional layer of anxiety, as we get obsessed with creating the perfect external conditions for sleep and then convince ourselves that we won't be able to sleep if those conditions are lacking. Remember, these are all just suggestions, so please don't place too much importance on them.

Turn Down the Lights

We are programmed both psychologically and physiologically to associate darkness with sleep. We need darkness to trigger the production of melatonin, the naturally tranquillizing hormone responsible for setting our sleep–wake pattern, but, alas, many of our evenings are spent peering at blue-light-emitting screens (laptops, tablets, phones), which stop this melatonin production. Just an hour of reading on an iPad delays melatonin release by two to three hours and disrupts the REM sleep in the following sleep cycle. In fact, artificial blue light actually triggers production of cortisol too, so try not to look at anything with a bright LED screen for at least an hour before bed. Start to dim the lights an hour or two before bedtime and keep your bedroom as dark as possible.

Also, be careful of those bright standby lights on TV sets and definitely make sure your smartphone is switched off or in airplane mode with the screen brightness turned down low.

Conversely, when you get out of bed and are ready to start your day, try to intentionally expose yourself to light. Sunlight is full of blue-spectrum light and when we wake up that's exactly what we want. Direct sunlight also helps to produce vitamin D, which is strongly linked to sleep health, and serotonin (the wakefulness hormone), which, in relation to melatonin production later on, is also highly beneficial for our wake–sleep cycle.

There are light receptors in your eyes that send information to the brain telling it to produce serotonin, so just gazing out of the window, even if it's overcast, will help tell the brain that it's time to wake up.

You can buy special Seasonal Affective Disorder light boxes for this, but natural light is often even better, as even on a cloudy day there is more benefit from 30 minutes of natural light than from hours in front of a light box.

Essentially, go dark before sleep and go bright when you wake.

~ *Sleep Notes* ~

Red light exposure can be quite good before bed, as it mimics melatonin-inviting firelight. Red light bulbs or candlelight can create this effect. I have a red LED lamp that I light my apartment with two hours before I intend to go to sleep and I try and brush my teeth by candlelight for maximum melatonin production before bed.

Keep Cool

In his audio book *The Yoga of Sleep*, Dr Rubin Naiman explains how insomnia is largely a disorder of body heat. When the sun goes down, the Earth cools, and human bodies are designed to do the same.

People with insomnia are often simply sleeping in rooms that are too warm (set a maximum bedroom temperature of 20°C/68°F; lower is even better). Alternatively, they may not have dissipated enough of their body heat energy during the day.

This overheating of our body is often exacerbated by our brain being too hot and energized too, which leads to excessive mental energy. In order to cool down, aim to reduce your consumption of light, processed food and processed information (including social media) before bedtime.

If you can, intentionally increase your energy output during the day by exercising more, but not within three hours of when you intend to go to bed. An Oregon University study found that you could improve your sleep quality by 65 per cent by getting two-and-a-half hours of moderate to vigorous exercise each week,[1] so exercise comes highly recommended.

If you are physically tired, sleep will come more easily to your body, but exercise also helps to quiet the mind as your brain will be less charged up with adrenaline than usual.

Don't Forget to Rest

Rest is the bridge from waking to sleep, yet so many of us try to skip over the bridge and end up lying in the darkness of racing thoughts before the hypnagogic even begins to set in.

Far better to create and cross that bridge intentionally before bed by doing 10 minutes or more of Yoga Nidra or a breathwork practice such as Coherent Breathing or the 4,7,8 Breath.

Hot baths are also a great way to create the conditions of rest and relaxation, as well as to cool down. A hot bath actually causes your body temperature to drop once you get out of it, creating the perfect conditions for sleep to follow.

Research has shown that a hot bath prior to bed can induce 15 per cent more restorative deep sleep in the sleep that follows too.[2]

Recreational reading before sleep can also help us rest before bed. Scientists at the University of Sussex have found that reading for just six minutes cuts stress levels by up to 68 per cent and that by reading you are 'actively engaging the imagination, as the words on the page stimulate your creativity and cause you to enter what is essentially an altered state of consciousness'.[3]

Talking of altered states, having a drink (or a smoke) before bed may seem to foster a state of rest, but let's not confuse sedation with relaxation. A glass of wine with your dinner will be metabolized out of your system within two or three hours, so don't worry about that; it's heavy drinking that we need to be cautious of, because going to bed drunk may help us fall into light sleep, but it tends to rob us of some of the REM and deep sleep that follows.

As for smoking, neither tobacco nor cannabis are very good for sleep, as nicotine is a stimulant and the THC in cannabis makes our REM periods shorter. The CBD compound in cannabis can be very helpful for relaxation, though, and doesn't have adverse effects on sleep, so CBD oil before bed may be helpful for many.

Sort Out Your Bedroom

First, try and eliminate noise, make it dark and get a bed that's comfortable. It may not be possible to get rid of all sound and light, but earplugs and blackout blinds can help. They are pretty inexpensive and will be well worth the money.

As for sound, the easiest stage of sleep to be roused from by noise is light sleep, and since we spend 50 per cent of our sleep time in that state, noise reduction becomes paramount. I had to try dozens of pairs of earplugs before I found ones that really worked for me.

~ Sleep Notes ~

The test for foam earplugs is called the springback test: squeeze the foam earplug between your fingers and release. The longer it takes to spring back to its full form, the denser the foam and the more noise reduction it offers. The best disposable foam earplugs I have found are called Hearos – Xtreme Protection Earplugs.

As for your bed, one of my best life tips is to get a comfy bed and comfy shoes, because if you're not in one, you're probably in the other. And yet the number of people who have a bed they don't like is astonishing. If you are strapped for cash, a thick mattress topper can transform even the most worn-out mattress for a fraction of the price of a new one.

Secondly, your sleeping space needs to support the *release* of energy rather than the creation of it. If possible, the bed should be used only for sleeping and sex, not for work. The bedroom should not look like a living room with a bed in it, or, even worse, an office with a bed in it. With so many more people working from home nowadays, this can be difficult to achieve, so don't stress over it too much, but at least try to make sure that your bed doesn't look like an office by the time you want to go to sleep in it.

Also, electronic wiring emits electromagnetic fields (EMFs), which have been shown to suppress the release of melatonin and stop some particularly sensitive people from becoming drowsy.[4] So, if you think you might have a particular sensitivity to EMFs, move anything with electronic wiring in it at least an arm's length away from your head.

And finally, try make yourself feel as safe as possible. It may help to go and double-check the locks on your front door. For people working with trauma, especially those who have experienced childhood sexual trauma, getting a simple lock fitted on the bedroom door can have hugely beneficial effects.

Be Coffee Smart

Coffee is generally a no-no in books about sleep, as it can reduce the amount of deep sleep that we have and having it within six hours of bedtime can actually reduce total sleep time by one hour.[5]

I think we need to look at this subject in a slightly more realistically way when working with trauma-affected sleep, though. For some people, a cup of coffee is a necessary evil to kick-start their day after a night of insufficient sleep and a welcome treat after a night of struggle, so let's look at how you can have coffee in the least worst way.

Caffeine has a half-life of about five hours. A half-life is the time it takes for our body to eliminate half the drug, so a 9 a.m. coffee should be out of our system by 7 p.m., but a 2 p.m. coffee will only have been fully metabolized by midnight.

It takes the bodies of older adults longer to process caffeine, though, so bear that in mind too.

Basically, try to avoid coffee after lunchtime if you can, but it's not a disaster if you can't.

Also, caffeine is habit-forming, meaning you will develop a tolerance to it if you have it regularly, so it is far better to use it strategically. If you only have a cup of coffee twice a week, when you do have it, you will be supercharged, whereas if you have several cups a day, it may not even register on your waking-state alertness and yet still play havoc with your sleep at night.

And finally, keeping regular sleeping hours comes highly recommended, but I've found that for people working with trauma, this can create just one more pressurizing expectation, so give yourself some slack on that one.

Remember, sleep is primarily governed by the state of the autonomic nervous system, so it's far more important to put your efforts into regulating that than stressing over the exact temperature of your bedroom and keeping the exact same sleeping hours.

Get your ANS in balance and you'll be able to relax deeply and sleep soundly in almost any conditions.

Notes and References

Introduction

1. The weather refers to what is happening at the moment, but the climate is the long-term environmental pattern of weather, which takes much longer to change, but once changed is often changed long-term. Catherine Duncan, a geographer I met on a Buddhist chaplaincy course, gave me this metaphor.

2. To read the full report, visit www.charliemorley.com/ wakeuptosleep [Accessed 24 June 2021]

3. American Sleep Association, 'Sleep and Sleep Disorder Statistics': www.sleepassociation.org/about-sleep/sleep-statistics [Accessed 24 June 2021]

4. Joe Rogan Experience #1109 (25 April 2018): Matthew Walker, www.youtube.com/watch?v=pwaWilO_Pig [Accessed 24 June 2021]

5. Krystal, A. (2008), 'The Treatment of Insomnia: New Developments': www.thedoctorwillseeyounow.com/content/ sleep/art1949.html [Accessed 24 June 2021]

Chapter 1: A Third of Our Life

1. Walker, M. (20 December 2017), 'Why We Sleep: Science of Sleep and Dreams', Talks at Google (20 December 2017): www.youtube.com/watch?v=aXflBZXAucQandt=1609s [Accessed 30 June 2021]

2. The National Sleep Foundation (NSF) says that the minimum requirement for adults is seven to eight hours: Chattu, V. K., et al. (2018), 'Insufficient Sleep Syndrome: Is it Time to Classify it as a Major Noncommunicable Disease?', *Sleep Science*, 11(2): 56–64.

3. Walker, op. cit.

4. Chaput, J. and Tremblay, A. (2012), 'Adequate Sleep to Improve the Treatment of Obesity', *CMAJ*, 184(18): 1,975–6.

5. Stevenson, S. (2016), *Sleep Smarter*. New York: Rodale Books, Introduction: xxviii.

6. Walker, op. cit.

7. Joe Rogan Experience #1109 (25 April 2018): Matthew Walker, www.youtube.com/watch?v=pwaWilO_Pig [Accessed 24 June 2021]

8. Ibid.

9. Loyola University Health System (2015), 'How Much Sleep Do we Need? Expert Panel Offers New Guidelines': www.eurekalert. org/pub_releases/2015-02/luhs-hms021115.php [Accessed 24 June 2021]

10. American Psychological Association (2014), 'More Sleep Would Make Most Americans Happier, Healthier and Safer': www.apa. org/research/action/sleep-deprivation [Accessed 24 June 2021]

11. American College of Cardiology (2014), 'Daylight Saving Impacts the Timing of Heart Attacks': www.acc.org/about-acc/press-releases/2014/03/29/09/16/sandhu-daylight-saving [Accessed 24 June 2021]

12. Ibid.

13. Mednick, S., et al. (2003), 'Sleep-Dependent Learning: A Nap Is as Good as a Night': https://pubmed.ncbi.nlm.nih.gov/12819785/ [Accessed 24 June 2021]

14. Walker, Joe Rogan Experience, op. cit.

15. American Psychological Association, op. cit.

16. Ibid.

17. Ibid.

18. Carter, A., et al. (2019), 'Mindfulness in the Military: Improving Mental Fitness in the UK Armed Forces Using Next Generation Team Mindfulness Training': www.researchgate.net/publication/337678323 [Accessed 24 June 2021]

19. Subjects who practised mindfulness meditation for just 30 minutes a day as part of a Massachusetts General Hospital study showed increases in grey-matter density of the hippocampus (an area responsible for learning and memory) and decreased density in the amygdala (an area responsible for anxiety and stress responses): Hözel, B. K., et al. (2011), 'Mindfulness Practice Leads to Increases in Regional Brain Gray Matter Density', *Psychiatry Research*, 191(1): 36–43.

20. William, C. (2017), 'Different Meditation Types Train Distinct Parts of Your Brain': www.newscientist.com/article/2149489 [Accessed 24 June 2021]

21. There is even a growing body of evidence to suggest that 'trauma can be fully integrated without cognitive awareness', although I would intuit that a body-based approach alongside psychotherapeutic talking therapy would probably be the ideal.

22. Cleveland Clinic (2020), 'Common Sleep Disorders': https://my.clevelandclinic.org/health/articles/11429 [Accessed 24 June 2021]

23. Ekirch, A. R. (2001), 'Sleep we Have Lost: Pre-Industrial Slumber in the British Isles', *American Historical Review* 106(2): 343–86.

24. Ekirch, A. R. (2016), 'Segmented Sleep in Preindustrial Societies': www.ncbi.nlm.nih.gov/pmc/articles/PMC4763365/ [Accessed 24 June 2021]

25. Hegarty, S. (2012), 'The Myth of the Eight-Hour Sleep': www.bbc.co.uk/news/magazine-16964783 [Accessed 30 June 2021]

26. Ekirch, 'Segmented Sleep in Preindustrial Societies', op. cit.

27. Beaumont, M. (2019), 'Insomnia and the Late Nineteenth-Century Insomniac: The Case of Albert Kimball': https://discovery.ucl.ac.uk/id/eprint/10095398/ [Accessed 24 June 2021]

Chapter 2: Knowledge Is Power

1.   Hegarty, S., (2012), 'The Myth of the Eight-Hour Sleep':
      www.bbc.co.uk/news/magazine-16964783 [Accessed 30 June
      2021]

2.   Everitt, H., et al. (2014), 'GPs' Management Strategies for
      Patients with Insomnia: A Survey and Qualitative Interview
      Study': https://bjgp.org/content/64/619/e112 [Accessed 24 June
      2021]

3.   Sleep scientists used to speak of five stages of sleep, but in 2007
      the American Academy of Sleep Medicine decided to group
      NREM3 and NREM4 together, making four stages.

4.   NIH Research Matters (2013), 'How Sleep Clears the Brain':
      www.nih.gov/news-events/nih-research-matters/how-sleep-
      clears-brain [Accessed 24 June 2021]

5.   Peters, B., 'How to Resolve a Lack of Deep Sleep': www.
      verywellhealth.com/lack-of-deep-sleep-3966027 [Accessed
      24 June 2021]

6.   WebMD (2019), 'Talking in Your Sleep': www.webmd.com/
      sleep-disorders/talking-in-your-sleep [Accessed 24 June 2021]

7.   Joe Rogan Experience #1109 (25 April 2018): Matthew Walker:
      www.youtube.com/watch?v=pwaWilO_Pig [Accessed 24 June
      2021]

8.   Walker, M. (2018), *Why We Sleep*. London: Penguin, p.208.

9.   Unless there is damage to the multimodal sensory cortex due to a
      stroke or head injury, and even then, after recovery, dreams will
      return.

10.   REM sleep behaviour disorder (RBD) occurs when subjects
      physically act out their dreams as they are dreaming them.
      When someone is woken from an episode of RBD, their dream
      description will usually fit with the physical movements that they
      were making, whether it's fighting off an attacker or smoking
      a cigarette. RBD in middle-aged men can often be a precursor
      to Parkinson's disease, and other subjects may have had their
      serotonin and dopamine levels upset by the use of antidepressant
      drugs such as serotonin-uptake inhibitors, which affect the

inhibition of motor systems during sleep. If you think you might have RBD, it's worth getting it checked out.

Chapter 3: Documenting Sleep: The Nocturnal Journal

1. Clive Holmes, a Buddhist teacher, once told me, 'Fear and fascination cannot exist within the mind at the same time.' When I first heard it, I thought it was surely too simplistic, but years later I still find it to be true.

2. For people who have PTSD or trauma, 50 per cent report having nightmares that exactly replay the trauma: Carr, M. (2016), 'Nightmares after Trauma: How Nightmares in PTSD Differ from Regular Nightmares': www.psychologytoday.com/gb/blog/dream-factory/201603/nightmares-after-trauma [Accessed 24 June 2021]

3. Walker, M. (2018), *Why We Sleep*. London: Penguin, p.204.

4. Walker, M. (2019), 'Why Do We Selectively Remember Dreams?': www.foundmyfitness.com/episodes/selectively-remember-dreams [Accessed 24 June 2021]

5. Arnulf, I., et al. (2014), 'Will Students Pass a Competitive Exam that they Failed in their Dreams?', *Conscious Cognition*, 29: 36–47.

6. Cocozza, P. (2018), 'Night Terrors: What Do Anxiety Dreams Mean?': www.theguardian.com/lifeandstyle/2018/oct/03/night-terrors-what-do-anxiety-dreams-mean [Accessed 24 June 2021]

7. For the full 'Mindfulness of Dream and Sleep' report, visit www.charliemorley.com/wakeuptosleep.

Chapter 4: Stressed-Out Sleep

1. Meadows, G. (2014), *The Sleep Book: How to Sleep Well Every Night*. London: Orion, p.32.

2. Elliott, S. B. (2005), *The New Science of Breath*, second edition. California: Coherence Publishing, 2005, p.8.

3. Brown, R. P. and Gerbarg, P. (2012), *The Healing Power of the Breath*. Trumpeter Books, p.10.

4. Ibid., p.34.

5. Email to the author, March 2021.

6. Stevenson, S. (2016), *Sleep Smarter*. New York: Rodale Books, p.14.

7. Cleveland Clinic (2021), 'Stress': https://my.clevelandclinic.org/health/articles/11874-stress

8. Davison, K. M., et al. (2020), 'Nutritional Factors, Physical Health and Immigrant Status Are Associated with Anxiety Disorders Among Middle-Aged and Older Adults: Findings from Baseline Data of the Canadian Longitudinal Study on Aging (CLSA)': www.mdpi.com/1660-4601/17/5/1493 [Accessed 24 June 2021]

9. Kim, T. D., et al. (2020), 'Inflammation in Post-Traumatic Stress Disorder (PTSD): A Review of Potential Correlates of PTSD with a Neurological Perspective': www.ncbi.nlm.nih.gov/pmc/articles/PMC7070581 [Accessed 24 June 2021]

10. Naiman, R., 'Mindful Sleep, Mindful Dreams' (blog): www.psychologytoday.com/us/blog/mindful-sleep-mindful-dreams/201101/how-cool-is-your-sleep

11. St-Onge, M.-P., et al. (2016), 'Fiber and Saturated Fat are Associated with Sleep Arousals and Slow Wave Sleep': https://jcsm.aasm.org/doi/10.5664/jcsm.5384 [Accessed 24 June 2021]

12. Davison, op. cit.

13. Littlehales, N. (2016), *Sleep*. Penguin Life: 2016, p.136.

Chapter 5: Hypnagogic Mindfulness

1. Organized by Sadaya, Keith McKenzie's veterans' charity.

2. Personal email from Uma.

3. Stankovic, L. (2011), 'Transforming Trauma: A Qualitative Feasibility Study of Integrative Restoration (iRest) Yoga Nidra on Combat-Related Post-Traumatic Stress Disorder': https://pubmed.ncbi.nlm.nih.gov/22398342/ [Accessed 25 June 2021]; iRest, 'iRest Yoga Nidra Research': www.irest.org/irest-research [Accessed 25 June 2021]

4. Pence, P. C., et al. (2014), 'Delivering Integrative Restoration-Yoga Nidra Meditation (Irest®) to Women With Sexual Trauma at a Veterans' Medical Center: A Pilot Study': https://pubmed.ncbi.nlm.nih.gov/25858651/ [Accessed 25 June 2021]

5. Ferreira-Vorkapic, C., et al. (2018), 'The Impact of *Yoga Nidra* and Seated Meditation on the Mental Health of College Professors', *International Journal of Yoga*, 11(3): 215–23.

6. Lou, H. C., et al. (1999), 'A 15O-H2O PET Study of Meditation and the Resting State of Normal Consciousness', *Human Brain Mapping*, 7(2): 98–105.

Chapter 6: Rest and Relaxation Practices

1. Hölzel, B. K., et al. (2011), 'Mindfulness Practice Leads to Increases in Regional Brain Gray Matter Density': www.ncbi.nlm.nih.gov/pmc/articles/PMC3004979/ [Accessed 25 June 2021]

2. Weir, K. (2016), 'The Science of Naps: Researchers are Working to Pinpoint the Benefits — and Possible Drawbacks — of an Afternoon Snooze': www.apa.org/monitor/2016/07-08/naps [Accessed 25 June 2021]

3. Donvito, T. (2020), '10 Things that Happen to your Body When you Take a Nap': www.thehealthy.com/sleep/benefits-of-napping/ [Accessed 25 June 2021]

4. Goldschmied, J. R., et al. (2015), 'Napping to Modulate Frustration and Impulsivity: A Pilot Study': www.sciencedirect.com/science/article/abs/pii/S0191886915003943 [Accessed 25 June 2021]

5. Fry, A. (2020), 'Napping': www.sleepfoundation.org/articles/napping

6. Mednick, S., et al. (2003), 'Sleep-Dependent Learning: A Nap Is as Good as a Night': https://pubmed.ncbi.nlm.nih.gov/12819785/ [Accessed 25 June 2021]

Chapter 7: Trauma and PTSD

1. In conversation with the author, November 2020.

2. Email from Dr Heather Sequeira to the author, April 2021.

3. In conversation with the author, November 2020.

4. For more information on her work, visit www. ptsdtraumaworkshops.co.uk/ [Accessed 25 June 2021]

5. Whalley, M. G., et al. (2013), 'An fMRI Investigation of Posttraumatic Flashbacks': www.ncbi.nlm.nih.gov/pmc/articles/ PMC3549493/#b0125 [Accessed 25 June 2021]

6. Kim, T. D., et al. (2020), 'Inflammation in Post-Traumatic Stress Disorder (PTSD): A Review of Potential Correlates of PTSD with a Neurological Perspective': www.ncbi.nlm.nih.gov/pmc/ articles/PMC7070581/ [Accessed 25 June 2021]

7. Cortisol has a neurotoxic effect on the hippocampus.

8. McGreevey, S. (2011), 'Eight Weeks to a Better Brain: Meditation Study Shows Changes Associated with Awareness, Stress': https:// news.harvard.edu/gazette/story/2011/01/eight-weeks-to-a-better-brain/ [Accessed 25 June 2021]

9. Williams, C. (2017), 'Different Meditation Types Train Distinct Parts of your Brain': www.newscientist.com/article/2149489-different-meditation-types-train-distinct-parts-of-your-brain/ [Accessed 25 June 2021]

10. Ibid.

11. Williams, op. cit.

12. Rendon, J. (2015), 'How Trauma Can Change You – For the Better': www.time.com/3967885/how-trauma-can-change-you-for-the-better/ [Accessed 25 June 2021]

13. Hefferon, K., et al. (2009), 'Post-Traumatic Growth and Life-Threatening Physical Illness: A Systematic Review of the Qualitative Literature', *British Journal of Health Psychology*, 14(2): 343–78.

14. Bloom, L. and Bloom, C. (2016), 'Post Traumatic Growth: The Benefits of Stress': www.psychologytoday.com/gb/blog/stronger-the-broken-places/201610/post-traumatic-growth

15. Rendon, op. cit.

Chapter 8: And Breathe…

1. Agarwal, D., et al. (2020), 'Equanimity in the Time of COVID: The Past Ameliorates the Present': www.ncbi.nlm.nih.gov/pmc/articles/PMC7456456/ [Accessed 30 June 2021]

2. Cromie, W. J. (2002), 'Meditation Changes Temperatures: Mind Controls Body in Extreme Experiments': https://news.harvard.edu/gazette/story/2002/04/meditation-changes-temperatures/ [Accessed 30 June 2021]

3. Brown, R. P. and Gerbarg, P. (2012), *The Healing Power of the Breath*. Trumpeter Books, p.35.

4. Philippot, P. (2002), 'Respiratory Feedback in the Generation of Emotion', *Cognition and Emotion*, 16(5): 605–627.

5. Nestor, J. (2020), *Breath: The New Science of a Lost Art*. London: Penguin Life, p.xvii.

6. In conversation with the author, January 2021.

7. Nestor, op. cit., p.6

8. Ibid., p.50

9. Ibid.

10. Tsubamoto-Sano, N., et al. (2019), 'Influences of Mouth Breathing on Memory and Learning Ability in Growing Rats': https://pubmed.ncbi.nlm.nih.gov/30918208/ [Accessed 30 June 2021] When this study's researchers explored the effects of mouth breathing on human subjects, they found a link to both sleep disorders and ADHD, caused by the imbalanced oxygen levels in the prefrontal cortex that mouth breathing creates.

11. Nunez, K. (2021), 'What Are the Advantages of Nose Breathing vs Mouth Breathing?': www.healthline.com/health/nose-breathing [Accessed 30 June 2021]

12. Baker, L. (2000), 'Lung Function May Predict Long Life or Early Death': http://www.buffalo.edu/news/releases/2000/09/4857.html [Accessed 30 June 2021]

13. Ibid.

14. Agarwal, op. cit.

15. Knutson, F. (2019), 'Why Watching the Breath Won't Work: HRV Breathing': www.youtube.com/watch?v=J_2A-m-oeQU&t=14s [Accessed 30 June 2021]

16. Ibid.

17. Ibid.

18. Ibid. The studies revealed that the average breath rate between 1929 and 1980 was six breaths per minute.

19. Whitworth, G. (2019), 'What is a Normal Respiratory Rate?': www.medicalnewstoday.com/articles/324409 [Accessed 30 June 2021]

Chapter 9: Coherent Breathing

1. Coherent Breathing is a registered trademark of COHERENCE LLC, founded by Stephen Elliott in 2005.

2. Awakened Mind, a trademark of the late Anna Wise, is used to describe a brainwave pattern that exhibits symmetrical amplitudes of brainwave bands delta, theta, alpha and beta in the Occipital Lobe 1 and Occipital Lobe 2 areas of the brain.

3. High heart rate variability (HRV) is a sign of good health. People with post-traumatic stress, anxiety or depression tend to have lower heart rate variability due to the dysregulation of their stress–response system. Coherent Breathing creates very high heart rate variability.

4. During an EEG study in which Richard Brown was hooked up to a brain scanner while he did Coherent Breathing, his brain went into such a deep state of alpha and theta brainwaves that they thought he was having a stroke and ended the experiment to check on him!

5. In conversation with the author, 2018.

6. Elliott and colleagues have documented an increase in alpha-brainwave amplitude with the first 'Coherent' breath that subjects took.

7. In conversation with the author, July 2020.

8. In conversation with the author, January 2021.

9.   Nestor, J. (2020), *Breath: The New Science of a Lost Art*. London: Penguin Life, p.83. Nestor mentions that the optimal breathing rhythm for most adults is actually about a five-and-a-half-second inhale followed by a five-and-a-half-second exhale, which then spookily works at works out at five-and-a-half breaths per minute! But anything between four and six breaths per minute will do the trick.

10.   The significance of 'resonance' is that it is the point where blood flow is the most effective and efficient. It is also the point where circulatory wave action is optimal.

11.   I am just under six feet tall, but I often prefer to breathe at 3.5 or 4bpm. This may be due to my fitness level being pretty high or my lung capacity already being pretty large. Work with what your body asks for, and if you want to slow down even more, feel free to do so.

12.   Nestor, op. cit.

13.   Something around a 'One Mississippi, two Mississippi, three Mississippi' pace will do, but if in doubt count slower rather than faster.

14.   In conversation with the author, January 2021.

Chapter 10: Breath–Body–Mind

1.   In conversation with the author, 2018.

2.   So much so that, in 2020, I became a certified teacher of it.

3.   In conversation with the author, July 2020.

4.   Bergland, C. (2016), 'Vagus Nerve Stimulation Dramatically Reduces Inflammation': www.psychologytoday.com/us/blog/the-athletes-way/201607/vagus-nerve-stimulation-dramatically-reduces-inflammation [Accessed 30 June 2021]

5.   Professor Stephen Porges, of polyvagal theory fame, discovered that slow, deep breathing was the easiest way to stimulate the vagus nerves other than internal electrical stimulation.

6.   Carter, J. J. and Byrne G. G. (2012), 'PTSD Australian Vietnam Veterans: Yoga Adjunct Treatment, Two RCTs: MCYI and SKY', National Academies Press, 13 July.

Chapter 11: Nightmares

1. As if mirroring the *Tibetan Book of the Dead*'s claim that 'Every week on the same day that death occurred, the dead being will die once more.'

2. Havens, J., (2018), 'Planned Dream Intervention Research Paper – Accepted Manuscript': www.researchgate.net/publication/330193927 [Accessed 30 June 2021]

3. In conversation with the author, August 2016.

4. Carr, M. (2016), 'Nightmares After Trauma: How Nightmares in PTSD Differ from Regular Nightmares': www.psychologytoday.com/gb/blog/dream-factory/201603/nightmares-after-trauma [Accessed 30 June 2021]

5. Carr, M. (2014), 'What's Behind Your Recurring Dreams? Why Dreams Generated by Long-Ago Stress Can Keep Coming Back': www.psychologytoday.com/gb/blog/dream-factory/201411/whats-behind-your-recurring-dreams [Accessed 30 June 2021]

6. In conversation with the author, July 2020.

7. Walker, M. (2018), *Why We Sleep*. London: Penguin, p.211

8. Anwar, Y. (2011), 'Dream Sleep Takes Sting Out of Painful Memories': https://news.berkeley.edu/2011/11/23/dream-sleep/ [Accessed 30 June 2021]

9. Valli, K., et al. (2005), 'The Threat Simulation Theory of the Evolutionary Function of Dreaming: Evidence from Dreams of Traumatized Children': https://pubmed.ncbi.nlm.nih.gov/15766897/ [Accessed 30 June 2021]

10. Antti Revonsuo in *Horizon* (2009): 'Why Do we Dream?', BBC Television.

11. Quoted in Walker, 'Dream sleep takes sting out of painful memories', op. cit.

Chapter 12: Night Terrors and Sleep Paralysis

1. This lack of narrative memory seems to be because the neurons in the neocortex (the brain's centre for higher mental functions) are less active in deep sleep.

2. Although this usually freaks parents out more than the children themselves, they're not usually a cause for concern. They are usually triggered by a maturing nervous system rather than underlying trauma, and usually pass as the child grows up.

3. Denis, D., et al. (2018), 'A Systematic Review of Variables Associated with Sleep Paralysis', *Sleep Medicine Reviews* 38: 141–57.

4. In conversation with the author, January 2021.

5. Ryan Hurd believes that this is why college students are more likely than almost any other group to experience occasional sleep paralysis – they are often both stressed out and not getting enough sleep.

6. In conversation with the author, January 2021.

Chapter 13: Nightmare Integration Exercises

1. Rinpoche, T. W. (1998), *The Tibetan Yogas of Dream and Sleep*. New York: Snow Lion Publications, p.102.

2. Roderik, J. S. G. and Band, G. P. H. (2018), 'Breath of Life: The Respiratory Vagal Stimulation Model of Contemplative Activity': www.ncbi.nlm.nih.gov/pmc/articles/PMC6189422/ [Accessed 1 July 2021]

3. Weil, A. (2016), 'Three Breathing Exercises and Techniques': www.drweil.com/health-wellness/body-mind-spirit/stress-anxiety/breathing-three-exercises/ [Accessed 1 July 2021]

4. Barrett, D. (1993), 'The Committee of Sleep: A Study of Dream Incubation for Problem Solving': www.researchgate.net/publication/254735243 [Accessed 1 July 2021]

5. Park, W. (2021), 'Why We Shouldn't Be Afraid of Nightmares': www.bbc.com/future/article/20210330-why-we-shouldnt-be-afraid-of-nightmares [Accessed 1 July 2021]

6. Most of us dream in visual images, so by creating a visual image of the dream, we provide a waking-state template for the subconscious mind to work with. This step of the process also helps to activate a brain region called the visual cortex – exactly the same brain region that is activated when we dream.

7. Renner, R. (2020), 'The Pandemic is Giving People Vivid, Unusual Dreams': www.nationalgeographic.com/science/article/coronavirus-pandemic-is-giving-people-vivid-unusual-dreams-here-is-why [Accessed 1 July 2021]

8. Ibid.

9. Sharma, V. K., et al. (2013), 'Effect of Fast and Slow Pranayama on Perceived Stress and Cardiovascular Parameters in Young Health-Care Students', *IJOY*, 6(2): 104–10.

10. André, C. (2019), 'Proper Breathing Brings Better Health': www.scientificamerican.com/article/proper-breathing-brings-better-health/ [Accessed 1 July 2021]

11. In conversation with the author, 2014.

Chapter 14: Making Friends with Monsters

1. Nunez, K. (2019), 'Lucid Dreaming: Controlling the Storyline of Your Dreams': www.healthline.com/health/what-is-lucid-dreaming#when-it-occurs [Accessed 1 July 2021]

2. A very powerful placebo effect can be engaged within a lucid dream and there are dozens of first-hand accounts of people healing physical health conditions through lucid dreaming.

3. The lucid dreaming practices found within Tibetan Buddhism are referred to as dream yoga. *Yoga* means 'union', and dream yoga is about unifying our mind within our dreams.

4. A 2011 study at Heidelberg University, Germany, and the University of Bern, Switzerland, concluded that 'lucid dreams have a great potential for athletes to use as a training method because lucid dreaming mimics a perfect simulation of the real world', but without the limitations of reality: Erlacher, D., et al. (2012), 'Frequency of Lucid Dreams and Lucid Dream Practice in German Athletes': www.researchgate.net/publication/230727513 [Accessed 1 July 2021]

5. Voss, U., et al (2009), 'Lucid Dreaming: A State of Consciousness with Features of Both Waking and Non-Lucid Dreaming', *Sleep*, 32(9): 1,191–1200.

6. Max-Planck-Gesellschaft (2012), 'Lucid Dreamers Help Scientists Locate the Seat of Meta-Consciousness in the Brain': http://www.sciencedaily.com/releases/2012/07/120727095555.htm [Accessed 1 July 2021]

7. Dresler, M., et al. (2011), 'Dreamed Movement Elicits Activation in the Sensorimotor Cortex', *Current Biology* 21(21): 1,833–7.

8. Erlacher, op. cit.

9. Zadra, A. L. and Pihl, R. O. (1997), 'Lucid Dreaming as a Treatment for Recurrent Nightmares': www.ncbi.nlm.nih.gov/pubmed/8996716 [Accessed 1 July 2021]

10. Ibid.

11. Ibid.

12. Spoormaker, V. I. (2006), 'Lucid Dreaming Treatment for Nightmares: A Pilot Study': https://pubmed.ncbi.nlm.nih.gov/17053341 [Accessed 1 July 2021]

13. European Science Foundation (2009), 'New Links Between Lucid Dreaming and Psychosis Could Revive Dream Therapy in Psychiatry': www.sciencedaily.com/releases/2009/07/090728184831.htm [Accessed 1 July 2021]

14. Mota-Rolim, S. A. and Araujo, J. F. (2013), 'Neurobiology and Clinical Implications of Lucid Dreaming': www.ncbi.nlm.nih.gov/pubmed/23838126

15. Freitas de Macêdo, T. C., et al. (2019), 'My Dream, My Rules: Can Lucid Dreaming Treat Nightmares?': www.ncbi.nlm.nih.gov/pmc/articles/PMC6902039/ [Accessed 1 July 2021]

16. A hug is a universal and archetypal symbolic expression of love and acceptance, and so if you can 'hug your monsters', as I explained in my 2011 TED talk, you have the potential to integrate trauma at a very deep level.

Chapter 15: Lucid Dream Practices

1. LaBerge, S. and Rheingold, H. (2009), *Exploring the World of Lucid Dreaming*. New York: Ballantine Books, New York.

2. Ibid.

3. Rinpoche, T. (2008), *Dream Yoga* (DVD), E-Vam Institute.

Conclusion

1. Morley, C. (23 April 2019), 'PTSD Treatment for Veterans', www.youtube.com/watch?v=GT70TiLFym4 [Accessed 1 July 2021]

Appendix

1. Oregon State University (2011), 'Study: Physical Activity Impacts Overall Quality of Sleep': https://synergies.oregonstate.edu/2011/study-physical-activity-impacts-overall-quality-of-sleep/ [Accessed 1 July 2020]

2. Horne, J. A. and Reid, A. J., 'Night-Time Sleep EEG Changes Following Body Heating in a Warm Bath': https://pubmed.ncbi.nlm.nih.gov/2578367/ [Accessed 1 July 2021]

3. 'Reading "Can Help Reduce Stress"' (2009), *Daily Telegraph*, 30 March.

4. Dyche, J., et al. (2012), 'Effects of Power Frequency Electromagnetic Fields on Melatonin and Sleep in the Rat', *Emerging Health Threats*, 5(1).

5. Drake, C., et al. (2013), 'Caffeine Effects on Sleep Taken 0, 3, or 6 Hours before Going to Bed': https://jcsm.aasm.org/doi/10.5664/jcsm.3170

Resources

I would like to invite you personally to connect with me on Instagram (Charlie_Morley_Lucid_Dreaming) or Facebook (Charlie Morley-Lucid Dreaming), as I always enjoy hearing from readers.

Even better would be to meet you either in person or online at a live workshop or at the free online Lucid Dream Drop-Ins that I run each month. The details for all of these can be found at www.charliemorley.com.

And here are some of my top recommendations for continuing your exploration of sleep and dreams.

'Mindfulness of Dream & Sleep' Workshops and Retreats

I continue to run 'Mindfulness of Dream & Sleep' workshops and retreats both online and in person.

My hope is that these will always be either free or greatly discounted for armed forces veterans and serving personnel.

I will also be releasing a 'Mindfulness of Dream & Sleep' pre-recorded online course based on many of the practices in this book in 2022.

See my website, www.charliemorley.com, for more information about both live workshops and online courses.

Lucid Dreaming Workshops and Sleepover Retreats

Learning lucid dreaming from a book is like learning to dance from a book: it is possible but it is nothing like going to an actual dance class. Those of you who want a more visceral experience might like to check out my lucid dreaming workshops and immersive sleepover retreats, which have so far taken place in over 20 countries around the world. Visit www.charliemorley.com for latest information.

If you want to go deeper into lucid dreaming and learn dozens of other induction techniques, you might like to check out my online courses and my other lucid dreaming books at www.charliemorley.com.

There are also loads of free videos on my YouTube channel: CharlieMorley1.

Shadow Integration Workshops and Retreats

I continue to run shadow integration workshops and retreats online and in person, and also have the 'Embracing the Shadow' online course available.

Shadow integration is a process of psychological transformation that helps us to turn shame into acceptance and fear into love. It is pretty powerful stuff, and my third book, *Dreaming Through Darkness*, explores this topic in depth.

See my website www.charliemorley.com for more information.

Recommended Organizations

Forward Assist Veterans' Charity: www.forward-assist.com

Kagyu Samye Dzong, London: www.london.samye.org

The Mindfulness Association UK: www.mindfulness association.net

PTSD Trauma Workshops: www.ptsdtraumaworkshops.co.uk

Sadaya Veterans Charity

Safely Held Spaces: www.safelyheldspaces.org

Samye Ling Tibetan Buddhist Monastery: www.samyeling.org

Veterans' Yoga Project: www.veteransyogaproject.org

Winston Churchill Memorial Trust: www.wcmt.org.uk

Recommended Reading

Steve Biddulph, *Manhood*, Finch Publishing, 1995

Richard P. Brown and Patricia Gerbarg, MD, *The Healing Power of the Breath: Simple Techniques to Reduce Stress and Anxiety, Enhance Concentration and Balance Your Emotions*, Trumpeter Books, 2012

Pema Chödrön, *When Things Fall Apart: Heart Advice for Difficult Times*, Harper Non-Fiction; Thorsons Classics edition, 2005

Stephen B. Elliott, *The New Science of Breath*, second edition, Coherence Publishing, 2005

Matthew Green, *Aftershock: Fighting War, Surviving Trauma, and Finding Peace*, Portobello Books Ltd, 2016

Ryan Hurd, *Sleep Paralysis: A Guide to Hypnagogic Visions and Visitors of the Night*, Hyena Press, 2010

Forrest Knutson, *Hacking the Universe: The Process of Yogic Meditation*, CreateSpace, 2012

Stephen LaBerge and Howard Rheingold, *Exploring the World of Lucid Dreaming*, Ballantine Books, New York, 1990

Peter A. Levine, *Waking the Tiger: Healing Trauma*, North Atlantic Books, 2009

Nick Littlehales, *Sleep: Change the Way You Sleep with this 90-Minute Read*, Penguin Life, 2016

Julie T. Lusk, *Yoga Nidra for Complete Relaxation and Stress Relief*, New Harbinger, 2015

Gabor Maté, *When the Body Says No: The Cost of Hidden Stress*, Vermilion, 2019

Dr Guy Meadows, *The Sleep Book: How to Sleep Well Every Night*, Orion, 2014

Dr Rubin Naiman, *The Yoga of Sleep: Sacred and Scientific Practices to Heal Sleeplessness*, audiobook, Sounds True, 2010

James Nestor, *Breath: The New Science of a Lost Art*, Penguin Life, 2020

Tenzin Wangyal Rinpoche, *The Tibetan Yogas of Dream and Sleep*, Snow Lion Publications, 1998

Shawn Stevenson, *Sleep Smarter: 21 Essential Strategies to Sleep Your Way to a Better Body*, Rodale Books, 2016

Bessel van der Kolk, *The Body Keeps the Score: Mind, Brain and Body in the Transformation of Trauma*, Penguin, 2015

Matthew Walker, *Why We Sleep: The New Science of Sleep and Dreams*, Penguin, 2018

Pete Walker, *Complex PTSD: From Surviving to Thriving*, Create Space Independent Publishing Platform, 2013

Jennifer Williamson, *Sleep Affirmations: 200 Phrases for a Deep and Peaceful Sleep*, Adams Media, 2018

Acknowledgements

There are so many people who deserve thanks and gratitude in regard to making this book happen.

Firstly, my teachers Lama Yeshe Rinpoche and Rob Nairn, both of whom have known trauma, nightmares and loss, and both of whom were courageous enough to be transformed by them. Everything in this book is inspired by their teachings.

Secondly, I'd like to thank Keith McKenzie, the man who started me out on the path of working with veterans and the military.

Huge thanks to Sunil, Kev, Keith, Cal, Lt. General Rob Magowan and all those at the Defence Buddhist Network whose consistent support over the past five years has helped me so much.

Thanks to the Winston Churchill Memorial Trust for the fellowship grant, and to all those who featured in the documentary, including Cliff Grady, Leo Joslin, Nick Mutafis,

Stephanie Lopez, and Dan and Perry from the Veterans' Yoga Project.

Thanks to all the amazing veterans from the Samye Ling Veterans' Mindfulness Retreats, including Tommy Addison, Matt Deeming, Byran, Chris Dunlop, Johnny Cashman and to brilliant teachers Penny Horner, Bill Paterson and squadron leader Fi Thompson.

Thanks to Tony and Paula from Forward Assist, and to James Scurry from Safely Held Spaces. Thank you to Zia Alley for the lockdown writing sessions and the check-ins during my darkest times. Thanks to the amazing Chris Lavin (Dynamic White Stag) and the brothers from the Mankind Project.

Thanks to Mantis Clan and Waffles, Tim the therapist and all those who helped me remember myself after that year of ego dismemberment. Thank you to that moment of rock bottom for showing me what I had to live for.

Thanks to all those whose work features in the book, including Dr Heather Sequeira, Uma Dinsmore-Tuli, Dr Richard Miller, Stephen Elliott, Dr Patricia Gerbarg and Dr Richard Brown, Dr Michelle Carr, Ryan Hurd and Justin Havens.

Thanks to all those who offered the 'Field-Tested Feedback' and to the lucid dreaming case studies of Ivan, Fiona, Robert and Ahmed (although the name has been changed, your soul remains in the story, brother).

Thanks to Ya'Acov Darling Khan and Tim Freke for opening the door to Hay House, and to Michelle Pilley for letting me in. Thanks to Lizzie Henry for the tireless editing work and to Jo, Julie, Rachel, Alexandra, Leanne, Diane, Susie, Katherine, Tom, Portia, Lizzi and the rest of the brilliant team at Hay House for all their hard work on the project.

Thanks to Jade, my mum, brother, dad and ancestors.

And thanks to all those who have walked with me on the road less travelled.

Charlie Morley
Summer Solstice 2021

ABOUT THE AUTHOR

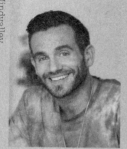

Mindvalley

Charlie Morley is a bestselling author and teacher of lucid dreaming, shadow integration and Mindfulness of Dream & Sleep.

He has been lucid dreaming for over 20 years and was 'authorised to teach' within the Kagyu school of Tibetan Buddhism by Lama Yeshe Rinpoche in 2008. Since then his books have been translated into more than 15 languages and he has run workshops and retreats in more than 20 countries.

Charlie has spoken at both Oxford and Cambridge Universities and has presented his findings on Mindfulness of Dream & Sleep at the Ministry of Defence Mindfulness Symposium. In 2018 he was awarded a Winston Churchill Fellowship grant to research PTSD treatment in military veterans, and continues to run workshops and retreats for people with trauma-affected sleep.

Charlie is a qualified teacher of both Yoga Nidra and Breath-Body-Mind, and has been the lead consultant on scientific studies into lucid dreaming for treatment of nightmares and PTSD at Swansea University Sleep Lab and the Institute of Noetic Sciences.

In his past life he trained and worked as an actor and scriptwriter before running a hip-hop dance collective throughout his 20s.

When he's not teaching he enjoys kickboxing, surfing and pretending to meditate.

www.charliemorley.com

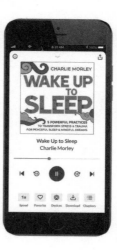

HAY HOUSE

Look within

Join the conversation about latest products,
events, exclusive offers and more.

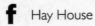 Hay House

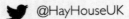 @HayHouseUK

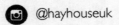 @hayhouseuk

We'd love to hear from you!